Foreword

Sudhir Srivastava
Cancer Biomarkers Research Group, National Cancer Institute, Bethesda, MD 20892, USA
Editor in Chief

The NCI's Early Detection Research Network (EDRN) structure and function provide a unique approach to translational research that is not readily accomplished through other mechanisms. The structure engages highly successful, independent, academic, peer reviewed scientists in a process of discovery and validation that requires deep collaboration. The EDRN attracts excellent academic and industry scientists by providing access to diverse top-quality scientific (assays), clinical specimens, methodological expertise, industrial resources, and financial resources that are not organized or are not readily available through other governmentally based or industry based funding mechanisms. The collection of abstracts from its 4th Annual Workshop held in Philadelphia from 20–22 March 2006, speaks for the diversity of the approaches, technologies, and studies focused toward translating biomarkers into clinical application. Progress reflected through these abstracts testifies that the EDRN is successfully building and implementing a vertically integrated pipeline of biomarkers for cancer early detection and risk assessment.

EDRN is also addressing an important "culture challenge" that is inherent to the academic system. The current system emphasizes individual achievement over collaborative work. For biomarker discovery and validation the current academic system is fragmented and unlikely to succeed. While these culture barriers have caused delays and slowed progress, a collaborative environment of scientific innovation linked to excellence in translational research is emerging. The work of growing a cohesive culture of sharing remains on track. Investigators continue to see the EDRN as a place wherein the products of this research can be brought for validation and generalization. Investigators have fully engaged the EDRN resource, generating extensive collaborative research, opening the pathway to translation of innovative technologies to validation and generalization to the public. Consequently, the EDRN's portfolio of biomarkers is now expanding as indicated in the number of abstracts presented in the meeting.

Cancer Biomarkers 2 (2006) 179–217
IOS Press

Poster Abstracts

Biomarker Discovery and Validation for Patient Selection Using Microdissected Tumor Tissues

Brian M. Balgley
Calibrant Biosystems, Gaithersburg, MD, USA

Calibrant Biosystems has developed a novel proteome platform to enable the combined, reproducible profiling and quantification of thousands of proteins in microdissection-procured tissue samples, including freshly frozen tissues and archived formalin-fixed and paraffin-embedded tissue collections. Proteome display results enabling patient discrimination from targeted brain and breast tumor tissues, along with validation by IHC and Western blotting of selected protein biomarkers, are shown.

Haptoglobin- A Potential Serum Tumor Bio-Marker in Small Cell Lung Cancer

Sohiya Yotsukura, Vaibhav Sachdev, Ravi Salgia and Ajit Bharti
Department of medicine, Boston University School of Medicine, Boston, MA, USA

Lung cancer is the leading cause of cancer death both in men and women in United States and a similar trend is seen in many other countries. The survival of the majority of lung cancer patients is less than two years. Lack of early diagnosis is one of the primary reasons for the high mortality rate. A number of biomarkers have been evaluated in lung cancer patients, however, their specificity and early stage diagnostic values are limited. Using traditional protein chemistry and proteomics tools, we were able to determine differential serum levels of haptoglobin in small cell lung cancer (SCLC). Quantitative estimation of serum haptoglobin in SCLC patients representing different disease stages were determined by immunoblott analysis using anti-haptoglobin. Three-fold higher serum haptoglobin was recorded in patients with SCLC (mean relative level of α-haptoglobin 2.98 ± 0.47) than those observed in the normal controls (mean relative level 1.0 ± 0.31), and was 2.06-fold higher than patients with no evidence of disease post-therapy (mean relative level 1.45 ± 0.32).The levels of α-haptoglobin in serum from patients with LD-SCLC and ED-SCLC were 2.25 ± 0.69 ($P < 0.005$) and 3.61 ± 0.57 ($P < 0.001$) respectively, both highly statistically significant when compared to the healthy subject control.

The acute phase protein haptoglobin (Hp) is a tetrameric structure joined by disulphide linkages among two α and 2 β chains. Based on the length of α-chains there are three isoforms of Hp; Hp1-1, 2-1 and 2-2. All isoforms have the same 243 amino acid β chain (2 in each isoform), approximately 40 kDa. Hp1-1 contains two identical α-1 chains (83 amino acids, mol wt 9 kDa); Hp2-2 contains two α-2 chains 142 (142 amino acids 16 kDa), Hp2-1 contains one of each α-1 and α-2. Both α and β chains are glycosylated. Three genetic polymorphism and varied glycosylation status of haptoglobin provides significant heterogeneity. Using 2-D gel electrophoresis more than forty isoforms of haptoglobin have been identified. Haptoglobin expression profile in tissue and serum has been correlated with different disease conditions including cancer. Higher serum level of α-haptoglobin has been shown to bear diagnostic/prognostic value in ovarian cancer. Importantly in a recent study higher serum level of specific haptoglobin isoforms has been demonstrated in ovarian cancer. Our preliminary data, using 2-D gel followed by immunoblott analysis indicates differential expression of haptoglobin isoforms in SCLC serum samples. We are optimizing Hp purification by two different methods to micro-characterize differentially expressed isoforms to determine the diagnostic/prognostic value of specific isoform in SCLC patients.

Automated Peak Picking and Alignment of TOF-MS Data for Biomarker Discovery and Early Cancer Diagnosis

Christine Bunai[a], Dariya Malyarenko[a,b], Haijian Chen[a], Maureen Tracy[b], Eugene Tracy[a], Maciek Sasinowski[a,b], Richard Drake[c], Lisa Cazares[c], O. John Semmes[c], Michael Trosset[a], Dennis Manos[a] and William Cooke[a]

[a]*College of William and Mary, Williamsburg, VA, USA*
[b]*INCOGEN, Inc., Williamsburg, VA, USA*
[c]*Eastern Virginia Medical School, Norfolk, VA, USA*

Mass spectrometry is now a standard tool for protein biomarker discovery. Revolutionary MS hardware advancements provide unparalleled high-throughput protein/peptide analysis with high resolving power, sensitivity and dynamic range. However, coordinating protocols and equipment across several laboratories is crucial for this technology to become an important clinical diagnosis tool [1]. This comparison requires software tools to extract meaningful and in-depth information from these complex data sets. Unfortunately, advancements in those tools have lagged behind. To this end, we (at the College of William and Mary) have developed automated tools for analysis of TOF-MS protein profiles using the VIBE-MS platform in conjunction with our colleagues at Incogen and Eastern Virginia Medical School (EVMS).

Here, we present our deconvolution [2], automated peak picking, and alignment procedures for processing large raw data sets from clinical samples of blood sera. We illustrate these procedures by the analysis of two SELDI-TOF data sets, both collected by EVMS as part of an Adult T-cell Leukemia study. Because the data sets were collected at different times (separated by 16 months) and have significantly different calibration parameters, they serve as a model for the combination of sets from different laboratories. Previous attempts to combine data from disparate laboratories have depended on aligning calibration peaks [3], but our approach uses a fully automated peak picking algorithm based on a maximum likelihood approach, and an alignment procedure based on direct "self calibration" of all peaks in the time domain. We will demonstrate an effective merging of the two data sets for direct comparison and an improvement by an order of magnitude in the mass precision for these data sets, compared to the standard analysis provided by the manufacturer.

References

[1] O. John Semmes et al., *Clinical Chemistry* **51**(1) (2005), 102–112.

[2] D.I. Malyarenko et al., *Clinical Chemistry* **51**(1) (2005), 65–74.

[3] A.J. Rail et al., *Proteomics* **5** (2005), 3467–3474.

TMPRSS2:ETV4 Gene Fusions Define a Third Molecular Subtype of Prostate Cancer

Scott A. Tomlins[a,1], Rohit Mehra[a], Daniel R. Rhodes[a,b,1], Lisa R. Smith[a], Diane Roulston[a], Beth E. Helgeson[a], Xuhong Cao[a], John T. Wei[c,d,e], Mark A. Rubin[f,g], Rajal B. Shah[a,c,d,e] and Arul M. Chinnaiyan[a,b,c,d,e]

[a]*Department of Pathology, University of Michigan Medical School, Ann Arbor, MI, USA*
[b]*Program of Bioinformatics, University of Michigan Medical School, Ann Arbor, MI, USA*
[c]*Department of Urology, University of Michigan Medical School, Ann Arbor, MI, USA*
[d]*Michigan Urology Center, University of Michigan Medical School, Ann Arbor, MI, USA*
[e]*Comprehensive Cancer Center, University of Michigan Medical School, Ann Arbor, MI, USA*
[f]*Department of Pathology, Brigham and Women's Hospital, Harvard Medical School, Boston, MA, USA*
[g]*Dana-Farber Cancer Institute, Harvard Medical School, Boston, MA, USA*

EDRN Biomarker Development Lab, University of Michigan, Ann Arbor, MI, USA

While common in hematological and mesenchymal malignancies, recurrent gene fusions have not been well characterized in epithelial carcinomas. Recently, using a novel bioinformatic approach, we identified recurrent gene fusions between the 5'-untranslated region of *TMPRSS2* and the ETS family members *ERG* or *ETV1* in the majority of prostate cancers. In vitro evidence suggested that the androgen response elements (AREs) in the promoter region of *TMPRSS2* drive the over-expression of *ERG* or *ETV1*.

Here, we interrogated the expression of all *ETS* family members in prostate cancer profiling studies and identified marked over-expression of the ETS family member *ETV4* in two of 98 of cases. In one such case, we confirmed the over-expression of *ETV4* using quan-

---

[1] These authors contributed equally to this report.

titative PCR, and by rapid amplification of cDNA ends (RACE), quantitative PCR and fluorescence in situ hybridization (FISH), we demonstrate that the *TMPRSS2* (21q22) and *ETV4* (17q21) loci are fused in this case. Intriguingly, the fusion transcript consists of sequence ~ 8 kb upstream of the reported transcriptional start site of *TMPRSS2* fused to *ETV4*. This fusion would not contain the characterized AREs in the *TMPRSS2* promoter, but the marked over-expression of *ETV4* only in the presence of this fusion suggests that additional AREs or enhancer elements may be present upstream of *TMPRSS2*. This result defines a third molecular subtype of prostate cancer and supports the hypothesis that dysregulation of *ETS* family members through fusions with *TMRPSS2* may be an initiating event in prostate cancer development.

Standard Specimen Sets for Assessing Cancer Biomarkers in Women

Patrick Sluss[a], Joseph M. Moy[b], Steven J. Skates[c], Nora K. Horick[c], Anna M. Minihan[c], Donna M. Kemp[d], Jeffrey R. Marks[e] and Daniel W. Cramer[f]

[a]*Pathology, Massachusetts General Hospital (MGH), Boston, MA, USA*
[b]*Reproductive Endocrine Unit, MGH, Boston, MA, USA*
[c]*Biostatistic Center, MGH, Boston, MA, USA*
[d]*Research Blood Components LLC, Brighton, MA, USA*
[e]*Pathology, Duke University, Durham, NC, USA*
[f]*Department of Obstetrics and Gynecology, Brigham and Women's Hospital, Boston, MA, USA*

Sera accumulated from cancer cases prior to treatment are necessary for performing early validation studies on cancer biomarkers as are control specimens from persons without cancer; but collections with good description of demographics on subjects or normative data on other biomarkers are often lacking. Multiple (identical) sets of sera from healthy controls as well as sera obtained prior to cancer treatment from cases would be a valuable resource for initial assessment of a new biomarker. However, while healthy controls can electively donate 200–300 ml of blood to permit assembly of multiple individual aliquots, this is not feasible in cancer cases about to undergo treatment, thus pooling of specimens is the only realistic option in cases. The Partners/Southwestern Clinical Epidemiologic Center in conjunction with the Duke Biomarker Development Laboratory has constructed 275 standard specimen sets, each enclosed in a cylindrical container called a "goblet." The contents of the sets are described below:

1. 140 sets each containing 115 individually-barcoded plastic straws holding 0.3 ml of sera from 95 female control subjects (39 pre- and 56 postmenopausal women) and 20 straws that each contain 0.3ml of pooled control sera for assessing the coefficient of variation (CV) of the assay. These sets are useful when only control specimens are needed for studying female cancers other than breast, ovarian, or endometrial cancer.

2. 20 sets that contain 122 plastic straws including the 115 straws described in (1) plus 7 additional straws containing sera from pools that represent benign and malignant pelvic disease. These 7 pools were constructed from blood collected pre-operatively from premenopausal women with endometriosis or late stage non-mucinous ovarian cancers, postmenopausal women with benign serous tumors or early or late stage non-mucinous ovarian cancers, and all women with mucinous ovarian cancer or endometrial cancer.

3. 115 sets that contain 127 straws including the 122 described in (1) and (2) plus 5 additional straws containing sera from pools that represent benign, pre-invasive, and invasive breast disease. The 5 pools were constructed from blood collected prior to surgical resection from premenopausal women with benign breast disease, post-menopausal women with benign breast disease, women with DCIS unselected for age, premenopausal women with invasive breast cancer, and post-menopausal women with estrogen receptor positive invasive breast cancer.

Comparing the "mean" level of a new marker in diseased populations (estimated from the pooled specimens) in relation to the distribution in healthy controls will allow initial assessment of the performance of a new biomarker compared to standard markers (CA125, CEA, CA72.4, CA15.3, and CA19.9) measured in the sets as well as a precise measure of the CV of the new assay. Those markers performing as good or better than standard biomarkers would move to the next level of investigation with assessment in individual cancer cases. The sets are stored in liquid nitrogen at the NCI Fredericks facility. Investigators may request a specimen set by application through the EDRN website that requires investigators to briefly describe the basis for linking the assay to female cancer and to agree to post results on the website allowing a cumulative and comparative database on biomarkers in women to be developed.

Use of a Monoclonal Antibody Against Human Mucin 9 for Immuno-Histochemical Studies of Oviductin Expression in Fallopian Tubes and Serous Ovarian Cancer

Christopher P. Crum[a], David W. Kindelberger[a], Michael G. Zwick[b], Ward C. Tucker[b], Rachel Kravitz[b], Jacob Kagan[c], Patrick Sluss[d] and Daniel W. Cramer[e]

[a]*Department of Pathology, Brigham and Women's Hospital, Boston MA, USA*
[b]*Neoclone Biotechnology, Madison, WI, USA*
[c]*Cancer Biomarkers Research Group, National Cancer Institute, Rockville, MD, USA*
[d]*Department of Pathology, Massachusetts General Hospital, Boston, MA, USA*
[e]*Department of Obstetrics and Gynecology, Brigham and Women's Hospital, Boston, MA, USA*

Oviductin, also known as MUC9, is a newly-described product of the human Mucin family of genes that also includes CA 15.3 (MUC1) and CA125 (MUC16); and like CA15.3 and CA125, is a membrane-bound protein. The expression of oviductin is relatively well confined to the fallopian tubes and enhanced during estrus, suggesting it may play a role in gamete transport and fertilization. In view of the value of peripheral levels of mucins, like CA15.3 and CA125, in ovarian cancer detection as well as emerging evidence that dysplastic lesions within the Fallopian tubes may be the source of advanced serous cancers that quickly spread to the ovary and peritoneum, oviductin is of potential interest as an ovarian cancer biomarker. Although the human oviductin gene has been cloned, no monoclonal antibody against human oviductin is currently available commercially. The Partners/Southwestern Clinical Epidemiologic Center, in conjunction with Neoclone Biotechnology, have created monoclonal antibodies (mAb) against 13mer and 9mer peptide sequences predicted to be antigenic. We have performed initial immuno-histochemical studies on several of the created antibodies and identified one oviductin mAb showing good staining of epithelium of the Fallopian tubes and serous ovarian cancers. Our next step in this biomarker discovery effort will be to use the oviductin mAb to recover human oviductin protein from fresh lysates of serous ovarian cancers, which would allow creation of an ELISA for further Phase I studies.

Novel Strategies for MALDI-TOF Profiling of Low Abundance Proteins in Human Serum

Lining Qi[a], Lifang Yang[a], Rebecca Pitts[b], Xiangming Fang[c], Richard Drake[a] and O. John Semmes[a]
[a]*Center for Biomedical Proteomics, Eastern Virginia Medical School, Norfolk, VA, USA*
[b]*Bruker Daltonics Inc., Billerica, MA, USA*
[c]*GenWay Biotech, Inc., San Diego, CA, USA*

Introduction: Protein expression profiling has been applied in serum proteomic strategies for the identification of disease biomarkers. Specifically, the interrogation of serum from large patient populations using moderately high-throughput approaches with final analysis on surface enhanced laser desorption ionization-time of flight (SELDI-TOF) and matrix assisted laser desorption ionization-time of flight (MALDI-TOF) has yielded compelling results. However, many of the protein/peptide "biomarkers" are, or derive from, relatively high-abundant serum proteins. While not necessarily diminishing the potential diagnostic value of these proteins/peptides it would appear that the current approaches are limited to the higher abundance proteome.

Methods: We have developed automated high-throughput approaches for depletion and subsequent concentration of serum samples prior to analysis by mass spectrometry. The sample was subjected to depletion of abundant proteins using polycolonal avian IgY immunoaffinity step (Biomek 2000). After binding to the IgY depletion, $> 95\%$ of serum proteins by mass were removed. The depleted serum was then subjected to hydrophobic (HIC), immobilized metal affinity capture – cupper (IMAC-Cu2+) and weak cation exchange (WCX) magnetic beads to preconcentrate the IgY unbounded proteins (ClinProt). WCX and HIC affinity step were able to preconcentrate IgY unbounded proteins/peptides and improve resolution of depleted serum samples on UltraFlex MALDI-TOF/TOF.

Preliminary results: The amount of starting sample, different combination of matrix solvents, and analyte to matrix ratio were optimized for optimal expression profiling using a steel or Anchor chip plate. The WCX and HIC affinity step led to preconcentration of proteins/peptide unbound to IgY and improved the resolution of depleted serum samples on UltraFlex MALDI-TOF/TOF. Specific parameters for sample preparation were saturated CHCA in 0.5% TFA 1:1 ACN and H2O as the matrix and 9:1 WCX or C8 eluate/matrix ratio. There were only 15 peaks detected with regular QC serum at S/N = 6, SIT = 3% without any depletion step involved. After IgY depletion, and under the same conditions, there were 40 and 63 peaks detected with WCX and C8 affinity concentration steps respectively in the m/z range of 1 ~ 10 kDa following IgY depletion. Only one of the peaks overlapped with the regular QC serum profiling.

Serum Glycoprotein Biomarker Discovery for Prostatic Disease Using Differential Lectin Capture Strategies

E. Ellen Schwegler, Gunjan Malik, Michael Ward, Shamina Mitchell, O. John Semmes and Richard R. Drake
Center for Biomedical Proteomics, Eastern Virginia Medical School, Norfolk, VA, USA

Large-scale mass spectrometry based expression profiling studies of serum proteins has relied primarily on chemical affinity approaches to selectively enrich and fractionate samples. The goal of this study was to use a biological affinity; lectin capture approach combined with different pre-fractionation and mass spectrometry methods to increase the breadth of disease specific protein identifications. An inherent advantage to this approach is the current availability and low cost of multiple lectins with different carbohydrate binding specificities, thus allowing panels of lectins to be readily assessed. Also, many lectins have weak affinity for binding to major serum carrier proteins, thus providing a straightforward front-end fractionation step. Three cohorts of prostatic disease serum sample sets were obtained from the Virginia Prostate Center biorepository and stratified based on PSA levels, biopsy proven prostate cancer staging and benign disease. A panel of six lectins with known carbohydrate binding specificities was tested individually to differentially capture serum glycoproteins. A mixture of broad coverage lectins and more specific lectins for sialic acid and fucose residues were used. Lectin bound glycoproteins were separated by gel electrophoresis, and bands of interest were excised, trypsin digested and directly applied to MALDI-TOF/TOF (Bruker Daltonics) or LC-MS/MS instrumentation (Thermo Electron) for protein identification. Overall, each lectin profile produced both differences and redundancies in the identified gly-

coproteins. For each lectin tested, minimal amounts of serum albumin were bound, while capture or exclusion of immunoglobulin species was variable depending on the carbohydrate specificity of the lectin. In general, use of more specific lectins targeting fucose and sialic acid residues provided greater differential identification of potential glycoprotein disease biomarkers relative to broader mannose and glucose binding lectins. Combined use of lectins with broad specificity and less common sugar modifications provided more comprehensive coverage for biomarker discovery in each sample cohort. A proposed experimental outline incorporating automated analysis, improved identification strategies for potential biomarkers, serum fractionation and carrier protein depletion strategies using lectin profiling will also be presented.

Enhanced Detection of Low Abundance Human Plasma Proteins by Immunodepletion of 20 Abundant Proteins

Lynn A. Echan, Hsin-Yao Tang, Glenn C. Tan and David W. Speicher
The Wistar Institute, Philadelphia, PA, USA

Serum and plasma are promising sources for cancer biomarker detection because blood is thought to contain protein constituents from all cells in the body, and blood collection is minimally invasive. However, the complex nature of plasma, and the presence of a modest number of very abundant proteins at > 100 μg/ml levels makes it impractical to systematically detect low abundance cancer biomarkers using current two-dimensional protein profiling methods such as 2-D gels or LC/LC-MS/MS. We previously showed that removing six abundant plasma proteins efficiently removes about 85% of total protein from human serum or plasma and enhances detection of lower level proteins. However, even with Top 6 depletion, extensive multi-dimensional protein fractions are required to enable detection of a substantial portion of the proteins present in plasma at low ng/ml levels or less. To further optimize detection of low abundance cancer biomarkers and/or increase analysis throughput, it is highly desirable to remove the next most abundant proteins as well as the Top 6 proteins. To test the benefits of more extensive protein removal, we systematically evaluated major protein depletion of human serum and plasma using small and large formats of Sigma's recently developed ProteoPrep 20 Immunodepletion kit. Three critical parameters that affect biomarker discovery were evaluated, including: 1) the effectiveness of removing targeted major proteins, 2) the specificity of targeted protein removal, and 3) the effects of sample simplification on protein loading in down stream separations and enhanced low abundance protein detection using several alterative protein profiling methods. To determine the specificity of major protein removal, bound and unbound fractions were analyzed using 2-D gels and by 1-D SDS PAGE followed by cutting the entire lane into uniform slices for trypsin digestion and LC-MS/MS analysis. All 20 targeted proteins were detected in the bound fraction as expected as well as a few non-targeted proteins, although most non-targeted proteins were also detected in the unbound fraction as well. Overall, specificity and efficiency of protein depletion was similar to alternative immunoaffinity products. However, because these 20 proteins represent about 98% of the total protein, the depleted fraction from a far greater volume of original plasma could be separated by downstream methods with dramatically enhanced detection of low abundance proteins. In summary, depletion of 20 abundant plasma proteins effectively removes targeted proteins with minimal non-specific binding, thereby allowing >100-fold increases in plasma volume loads in most down stream analysis methods. As a result, more low abundance proteins can be detected by our 4-D protein profiling method or alternatively, similar depths of analysis can be obtained with less extensive fractionation and greater throughput compared with protocols that deplete less proteins.

Prevalence of High Level Overexpression of Candidate Biomarkers for Non-Small Cell Lung Carcinoma (NSLCLC) Confirmed by qRT-PCR

Wilbur A. Franklin, Jerry Haney, Lynne Bemis, Michio Sugita and John D. Mitchell
University of Colorado Health Sciences Center at Fitzsimons, Aurora, CO, USA

Biomarkers discovered through oligonucleotide microarray analysis must ultimately be validated by non-array methods. We have previously identified 20 genes that are highly overexpressed in lung carcinoma and have winnowed this list to 5 genes with properties that make them potentially useful biomarkers. Many of the biomarkers tested are members of the CTAG family of genes that are demethylated in carcinoma but are normally silent in all benign tissues but germ cells. In the present study, we used qRT-PCR to confirm the elevated levels of a promising subset of biomarker candidates in human lung cancers. To accomplish this we analyzed RNA extracted from 48 flash frozen NSCLC tumors and matched normal lung tissue. Four CTAG genes (MAGE A1-6, XAGE, NY-ESO and TEX15) and one non-CTAG candidate (PGP 9.5) were tested by a sensitive quantitative RT-PCR (qRT-PCR) method. Absolute RNA transcript copy numbers were determined from standards created by insertion of the target gene into TA vector and measurement of purified cDNA extracted from vector transfected bacterial cells. β-actin was used to normalize the amount of intact RNA available per sample and all results are reported as copies of biomarker transcript/10^6 copies of β-actin. ROC was used to calculate sensitivity and specificity of the various genes and to establish cutpoint levels for tumor. We found remarkable diversity in the levels of expression of these markers in benign lung tissue so that there were large differences in cutpoints among the markers. To achieve $p < 0.05$ between tumor RNA and benign lung tissue, cut points were set at 88 copies for MAGE, 1700 for XAGE, 1119 for NYESO, 80 for TEX15 and 155,000 for PGP 9.5. Using these cut points we found that 15% of NSCLC were positive for MAGE, 35% for XAGE, 0% for NY-ESO, 21% for TEX15 and 31% for PGP9.5. Overall, 69% of tumors were positive for one or more biomarkers. These results indicate that:

1. no single biomarker is likely to have sufficient sensitivity to be successful as a biomarker for early detection and prognosis
2. there is only partial overlap in the expression of the various CTAG markers
3. qRT-PCR is highly sensitive platform for detecting tumor associated RNA and could be directly applied to the detection of rare tumor cells in blood and other fluids
4. the upper limit of sensitivity for blood, sputum and urine assays for the combination of these five markers is likely to approximate 70%

Electrochemiluminescent Multiplexed Measurement of Biomarkers: Current Applications in Research and Future Applications in the Clinic

E.N. Glezer, J.D. Debad, A. Abdu and J.N. Wohlstadter
Meso Scale Diagnostics, Gaithersburg, MD, USA

As biomarkers gain a prominent role throughout drug discovery, clinical studies, diagnostics and therapeutic monitoring, they create a need for effective measurement in each setting. Desired attributes of systems for such measurements can include: 1) sensitive detection of biomarkers in various clinical samples, 2) the ability to measure multiple markers in a single sample, and 3) large detection range to simultaneously measure low- and high-abundance analytes. We describe two platforms developed by MSD to address these needs based on multiplexed electrochemiluminescent detection.

The first platform, developed for centralized high-throughput measurements, uses multi-well plates with integrated electrode arrays to perform up to 100 measurements per well at a rate of over 1000 data points per minute. MSD has applied this technology to sensitive, multiplexed biomarker immunoassays in serum and plasma samples. Assays have been developed for markers of inflammation, cancer, cardiovascular disease, endocrinology, fertility, and Alzheimer's disease. Many of these assays have been combined into multiplexed panels.

The second platform is currently being developed to address the needs of future Point-Of-Care clinical applications with multiplexed measurements on disposable cartridges. The fully self-contained cartridges are capable of performing up to 16 quantitative biomarker measurements on a few drops of whole blood, serum or plasma without sample processing. Results with sensitivities comparable to central laboratory analyzers are obtained within 15 minutes. Examples of multiplexed measurements of cardiac markers in human serum and whole blood will be presented.

Direct Biomarker Concentration Measurements in Serum Using Carbon Nanotube Capacitor Chips

Mikhail Briman[a], Erika Artukovic[a], David Chia[b,c], George Gruner[a,d] and Lee Goodglick[b,c]
[a]*Department of Physics, UCLA School of Medicine, CA, USA*
[b]*Department of Pathology and Laboratory Medicine, UCLA School of Medicine, CA, USA*
[c]*Johnsson Comprehensive , University of California, Los Angeles, CA, USA*
[d]*Cancer Center, California Nanosystem Institute at UCLA, University of California, Los Angeles, CA, USA*

The UCLA BRL in collaboration with the UCLA Department of Physics and the California NanoSystems Institute at UCLA is developing a novel high-density nanoscale device for direct electrical quantita-tion of tumor biomarker protein levels. This device is cost-effective to manufacture and use, and can be readily multiplexed to detect multiple antigens simultaneously. The design of this chip capitalizes on the quantum capacitance properties of single walled carbon nanotube networks. This nanoscale capacitor is highly sensitive to charge alterations at the surface of the nanotube/plastic platform. Here we present the first phase of this project, focused on proof-of-principal detection of a single representative biomarker, PSA. Monoclonal anti-PSA antibody was non-covalently absorbed onto the nanotube capacitor surface. Briefly, the assay set-up was as follows: a base-line reading is obtained with the carbon nanotube capacitor coupled to a reference electrode. The device is then incubated with serum for 30 minutes, rinsed with PBS, then capacitance is measured and compared to the base-line reading. Comparison with a calibration curve (calf serum plus 0–200 ng/ml recombinant PSA), determines the concentration of PSA in the serum sample. Addition of serum alone without PSA (i.e., either calf serum or serum samples from females), followed by rinsing, caused no change in capacitance above baseline levels.

Although the work presented here represent only the first phase of our development of this platform, there are a number of significant advancements that should be noted. This study represents the first direct electrical detection of biological markers from serum. Initial findings suggest that the level of sensitivity and specificity are comparable to standard techniques such as ELISA. Significantly, this platform has a number of advantages over conventional assays including direct detection, as a opposed to 'sandwich-type' assays, and virtually unlimited multiplexing capabilities (e.g., a cm^2 detection chip with numerous nanoscale capacitor subunits each with a unique antibody reagent).

Na,K-ATPase as a Cancer Biomarker: Implication in Cancer Progression and Prognosis

Sigrid Rajasekaran, Landon Inge, David Seligson, Sonali Barwe, Lee Goodglick, David Chia and Ayyappan Rajasekaran
Department of Pathology and Laboratory Medicine, David Geffen School of Medicine, University of California at Los Angeles, CA, USA

Na,K-ATPase also known as sodium pump consisting of α- and β-subunits is involved in maintaining intracellular sodium and potassium homeostasis in mammalian cells. The sodium gradient generated by Na,K-ATPase across plasma membrane is crucial for the various ion and metabolite transport across epithelial cells. Epithelial to mesenchymal transition (EMT) is one of the events associated with progression of cancer to a metastatic disease. During EMT epithelial cells loose their well-differentiated phenotype, gain motility and invasiveness. These properties of carcinoma cells underlie progression of cancer to metastatic disease. Understanding events that control EMT is crucial to development of therapeutic strategies. We show that Na,K-ATPase enzyme function and its subunits levels are affected in cells undergoing EMT. Repletion of sodium pump β-subunit expression in invasive carcinoma cells suppressed their motility and invasiveness and attenuated tumor forming potential in nude mice. Furthermore, RNAi mediated knockdown of β-subunit in well differentiate kidney epithelial cells induced a poorly differentiated phenotype indicating that this protein function is crucial for the structure and function of epithelial cells. Using tissue microarray technology we also provide evidence that Na,K-ATPase subunits levels predict recurrence and survival in bladder and kidney cancers respectively. Studies are on-going examining the expression and diagnositc/prognostic significance of Na, K-ATPase in lung, breast and prostate cancers using TMAs constructed by the UCLA BRLThese results highlight that Na,K-ATPase once considered as a house keeping protein has a potential value as a biomarker for cancer progression and prognosis.

The Use of Paraffin Embedded Tissues in Analyses Using Real Time Quantitative PCR[1]

Adam Steg[a], Martin Johnson[a], Wenquan Wang[b] and William E. Grizzle[c]
[a]*Department of Clinical Pharmacology, University of Alabama at Birmingham, AL, USA*
[b]*Department of Medicine/Biostatistics, University of Alabama at Birmingham, AL, USA*
[c]*Department of Pathology, University of Alabama at Birmingham, AL, USA*

In determining the aggressiveness of tumors and/or in predicting responses of tumors to specific therapies, many years can be saved by analyzing tissues removed several years previously and maintained as paraffin embedded tissues in archival collections. Although for some biomarkers, immunohistochemistry can be used for analysis of paraffin sections, for other biomarkers analysis by real-time–quantitative PCR (RT-Q-PCR) may be preferred. The effects of fixation and paraffin embedding, as well as long term storage of blocks, on analysis of mRNA extracted from paraffin sections have been uncertain. We evaluated gene expression using a novel TaqMan low density array of 26 and 20 genes in the hedgehog and Wnt pathways respectively. Specifically, we evaluated six frozen and mirror matched fixed paraffin embedded (FPE) tissues, each pair having the diagnosis of ovarian endometroid carcinoma. Expression values were normalized to uninvolved ovarian epithelium. The concordance between the results of expression of the same genes between frozen and FPE tissue was $r = 0.92, p < 0.0001$. Amplification of the mRNA from FPE tissues was not successful. TaqMan low-density assay provides an effective multiplex technique for examining gene expression based upon RNA isolated from archival FPE tissues.

[1]Supported in part by the Early Detection Research Network, William E. Grizzle, P.I. (5U24CA086359-06).

Genetic Profiling by Solid Phase Gene Extraction[1]

P. Scherp and K.H. Hasenstein
Biology Department, University of Louisiana, LA, USA

We developed a method for mRNA extraction and quantification that combines extreme sensitivity, fast sampling, high spatial resolution and minimal damage to tissue or even single cells. Solid Phase Gene Extraction (SPGE) in combination with quantitative real-time PCR is able to extract and quantify mRNA from rigid plant and soft animal cells. We present data illustrating that SPGE detects changes in gene expression in the same cell over time, quantifies high and low abundance mRNAs and localizes mRNA distributions in single *Drosophila* eggs. SPGE employs covalently bonded poly-T nucleotides to bind polyadenylated RNA to the surface of a micron-sized needle. Sampling results from inserting the probe into the tissue or cell of interest for less than one min. Using reverse transcription, cDNA is generated and used for further amplification. We used this novel approach to sample rigid algal cells, or a single *Arabidopsis* root tip multiple times without damaging the sampled cells or tissue. Using specific primers with quantitative real-time PCR quantified isoforms of high and low abundance actin, glucan-synthase and an auxin-induced gene. Application of hormones leads to detectable changes in mRNA expression in less than one hour. SPGE confirmed differential distribution of Nanos and Bicoid mRNA in less than four hour old Drosophila eggs. Nanos levels were five-times higher in the posterior than the anterior part of the egg; Bicoid was distributed evenly. Repeated sampling of the same cell as well as simultaneous sampling of the same cell at different sites illustrated changing mRNA patterns and corroborates SPGE's high spatial and temporal sensitivity and to-date the only technique that allows non-destructive sampling. We anticipate that further refinements of SPGE will result in fast, accurate, and simple diagnostic tests and enable genetic profiling of cancerous cells or tissue. Preparing (mixes of) gene-specific RNA templates may permit diagnosing specific states and combinations of malignancies.

[1]Supported by NASA grants NAG2-1423 and NAG10 -0190.

Printed Glycan Array Identifies Specific Signatures of Anti-Glycan Autoantibodies as Biomarkers in Sera of Breast Cancer Patients: Diagnostic, Prognostic And Therapeutic Opportunities

Margaret E. Huflejt, Ola Blixt, Marko Vuskovic, Hongyu Xu, James C. Reuben, Henry M. Kuerer and Massimo Cristofanilli
GlycoMedical Research Institute, La Jolla, CA, USA
Consortium for Functional Glycomics and The Scripps Research Institute, La Jolla, CA, USA
Computer Science, San Diego State University, San Diego State University, CA, USA
Departments of Breast Medical Oncology and Surgical Breast Oncology, UT M.D. Anderson Cancer Center, Houston, TX, USA

Background: Malignant transformation and tumor progression are associated with the specific changes in the complex surface carbohydrates, known as Tumor-Associated Carbohydrate Antigens (TACAs). TACAs are present in all human malignancies, however, little is known about the immune response to them. A printed glycan array containing many known TACAs and related glycans has been recently developed and validated. We have used this technology to simultaneously detect multiple anti-glycan autoantibodies in serum samples obtained from patients with metastatic (MBC) and primary breast cancers (PBC), in a search for biomarkers that represent a "breast-cancer-related signature" and therefore could be used as screening and diagnostic tools. We speculated that specific autoantibody profiles may be associated with early disease status or otherwise have prognostic implications.

Methods: A total of 57 serum samples from MBC (48%), PBC (26%) and healthy donors (26%) were analyzed. Glycan array slides were incubated with sera diluted with PBS/3% BSA, then with biotinylated goat antibody against human IgG, IgM and IgA, and with streptavidin-Alexa 488. The intensity of fluorescence in spots corresponding to the antibodies bound to the individual glycans was quantified with ImaGene image analysis software and data were plotted using MS Excel software.

Computational data evaluation: The univariate t-test and multivariate Hotelling's test were used to establish the significance in differences in anti-glycan autoantibody levels between "healthy controls" and breast cancer serum samples. To visualize data clustering, the Fisher-Rao projections, as well as projections based on support vector machines (SVM) were used.

Results and discussion: Breast cancer is associated with significantly higher levels of several autoantibodies against glycans including N-acetyllactosamines (LacNAc), fucosylated, and Core-2 glycans. Autoantibodies against 6-sulfo lactose, sialylated poly LacNAcs and O-linked T-antigen show most significantly increased levels in MBC as compared to PBC and healthy individuals.

Our studies demonstrate that the printed glycan array is a sensitive and promising tool for the identification of glycan-based cancer biomarkers, and for the development of clinical serum-based screening tests for early detection and evaluation of malignancy status. The unique method for defining clusters of circulating anti-glycan autoantibodies may lead to identification of specific TACAs as potential targets for the development of anti-cancer therapeutics.

Novel Domain-Specific Anti-MUC4 Antibodies: New Tools for the Diagnosis of Pancreatic Cancer

Maneesh Jain, Ganesh Venkatraman, Nicolas B. Moniaux, Michael A. Hollingsworth and Surinder K. Batra
University of Nebraska Medical Center, Omaha, NE, USA

Human MUC4 is a highly glycosylated membrane-associated mucin, which exhibits differential overexpression in pancreatic adenocarcinomas and is undetectable in the normal pancreas. MUC4 is a 930 kD glycoprotein that consists of two putative domains, namely, the large 850-kD sub unit, MUC4α, containing the identical 16 amino acid tandem repeat region and MUC4β, an 80 kD membrane-bound subunit, containing the cysteine rich domain, domain rich in N-glycosylation sites and three EGF-like domains. We have previously generated and characterized a MAb recognizing the tandem repeat (TR) region of the MUC4 protein, which has served as an important reagent in understanding the role of MUC4 pancreatic cancer. Using the anti-TR antibody a progressive increase in MUC4 expression has been observed in pancreatic intraepithelial neoplastic lesions. Functional studies from our group using anti-sense- and/or short-interfering RNA (siRNA) oligonucleotide-based and ectopic expression of MUC4 have provided substantial evidence of its role in the promotion of pancreatic tumor cell growth and metastasis *in vivo*. These observations suggest an intimate link between aberrant MUC4 expression and the pathogenesis of pancreatic cancer and it is believed that MUC4 can serve as an important serum marker for the diagnosis of pancreatic cancer. The anti-TR antibody can serve as a useful reagent for sensitive detection of MUC4 in serum as the highly repetitive nature of the TR (upto 400 times), provides multiple epitopes per molecule. However due to the high degree of polymorphism in the number and heavy glycosylation of TRs, the anti-TR antibody based quantitation can be inaccurate.

We report the generation and characterization of MAbs directed against various non-TR domains of MUC4. The N-terminal domain of MUC4α with and without the imperfect (126 aa) repeats upstream of TR region (MUC4αN-ter and MUC4αN-terR respectively), the C-terminal of alpha domain downstream of TR region (MUC4αC-ter) and MUC4β domains were cloned and expressed as GST-fusion proteins in *E. coli*. The purified proteins were used as immunogens for production of monoclonal antibodies, with alternate boosting with cell lysates expressing MUC4. We identified a number of positive clones exhibiting domain specific reactivity towards recombinant GST-fused MUC4 domains. No cross reactivity was observed with other recombinant MUC4 domains or with GST. In immunoblot analysis, two of the antibodies directed against MUC4α and one against MUC4β, exhibited similar reactivity towards MUC4 similar to that of the anti-TR antibody. All these three antibodies were capable of immunoprecipitating MUC4 from the pancreatic cancer cell lysates and reacted with the protein immunoprecipitated by anti-TR antibody. Specificity was further evaluated by laser scanning microscopy in MUC4-expressing vs. – nonexpressing pancreatic cancer cell lines. We conclude that, these domain specific antibodies could serve as useful reagents for developing *in vitro* MUC4 based serodiagnostic method(s) for detection of pancreatic cancer.

Use of Random Fine Needle Aspiration to Measure RNA Expression of Steroidogenic Enzymes in the Breast

S.A. Khan, D. Ivancic and T. Zaichuk
Robert H. Lurie Cancer Center of Northwestern University, Chicago, IL, USA

Random fine-needle aspiration (rFNA) is an efficient method of breast epithelial sampling which can be used to measure expression of specific gene sets. We are interested in the expression of steroidogenic genes in normal breast epithelium in order to define the local hormonal environment of the breast, since the importance of local estrogen production in the development and progression of breast malignancies cancer is increasingly recognized.

Methods: Epithelial cells were obtained by random fine-needle aspiration (FNA) of mastectomy samples. Twenty nine specimens of fresh-frozen FNA material were available for gene expression analysis. Total RNA was extracted by homogenizing cellular samples in 1 ml of TRIzol reagent (Sigma-Aldrich, St. Louis, MO) followed by a phenol-chloroform phase extraction and isopropanol precipitation. All of the RNA samples were treated with DNase and quantified by spectrophotometry. RNA samples were stored at $-80°C$ until they were processed for amplification and reverse transcription. The Full Spectrum RNA Amplification Kit (Systems Bioscience, Inc.) was used in the synthesis and amplification of cDNA. Real-time PCR was carried out with the 7900HT (Applied Biosystems, Foster City, CA) using Taqman primers and probes for the following panel of genes: estrogen receptors α and β (ERα, ERβ) steroid sulfatase (STS), aromatase (Cyp19), 17βhydroxy-steroid dehydrogenase types 1, 2, 5 (HSD1, HSD2, HSD5).

Results: Relative gene expression of ERα was low, and ERβ was high, as expected from normal breast tissue samples. No significant correlations were detected between the expression of ERα and other genes. ERβ expression on the other hand, demonstrated significant

Table 1

Pearson correlation coefficient between ERβ gene expression and expression of steroidogenic genes expressions in human breast cancer

Enzyme	Correlation coefficient	p value
STS	0.6285449	0.0007657
Cyp19	0.1150811	0.629
17HSD2	0.4989938	0.01536
17HSD5	0.6110067	0.001177
17HSD1	0.3773514	0.1835

Note: All values were log transformed to improve normality.

positive correlations with STS, the reductase enzyme HSD1 (promotes the formation of estradiol from estrone), and the oxidase enzyme HSD2 (metabolizes estrone to estradiol).

Conclusions: These results demonstrate that random FNA samples provide sufficient cell numbers and quantities of RNA to measure expression of multiple genes, and reveal meaningful relationships. They also highlight a potential new role for ERb in the regulation of steroid synthesis in the breast. These studies, when taken further, may allow the identification of women with specific steroidogenesis pathways in breast tissue, and therefore enable targeted interruption of these.

A Functional Genomic Approach to Biomarker Discovery in Pancreatic Cancer

Ann M. Killary, Marsha Frazier, Steven Lott, Jennifer Carter, David Stivers, Jane Chen, Rosa Hwang, James Abbruzzese and Subrata Sen
M. D. Anderson Cancer Center, University of Texas, TX, USA

We are pursuing a concerted genomics and molecular genetics approach to characterize putative target genomic loci implicated at high frequency in the genesis of pancreatic cancer. The chromosomal loci we are investigating include the target tumor suppressor gene(s) residing on chromosomes 1p and 3p and minimally amplified regions harboring putative oncogenes on chromosomes 20q and 12p, as well as, a novel oncogene Aurora-A/STK15 (Zhou et al., 1998) on chromosome 20q13.2, found amplified in a significant number of pancreatic cancers (Li et al., 2003) We hypothesize that pathways involving tumor suppressor genes with loss of function mutations/deletions and dominantly activated/amplified/over-expressed oncogenes are critical determinants in the development of early phases of pancreatic neoplasia

In the Killary lab, to identify chromosome 3p pathway genes we have identified 900 cDNAs from a subtraction hybridization library containing cDNAs differentially expressed between microcell hybrids with an introduced normal chromosome 3p12 fragment and which are suppressed for tumorigenicity in vivo and a 3p12 fragment-containing microcell hybrid which is deleted for a 2Mb interval and fails to suppress tumors in vivo. Since this library was originally developed in a system where the introduction of chromosome 3p mediated dramatic tumor suppression, all differentially expressed sequences represent genes that are in a pathway directed by a gene or genes present on the introduced normal chromosome 3. Characterization of this library will potentially aid in defining new genetic networks in pancreatic cancer. First pass sequencing of the library has been completed with 398 clones obtained from the suppression subtraction experiment selected for further analysis *in silico*. Initial BLAST analysis indicated that greater than one-third of the sequences analyzed correspond to either previously uncharacterized, hypothetical proteins, or alternative splice products. We believe that this kind of approach will complement the information that we obtain from screening the Affymetrix gene chip in terms of identifying genes that are differentially expressed in pancreatic tumor/normal samples. The marriage of the subtraction hybridization library gene information with the Affymetrix gene expression data will offer a unique resource for biomarker discovery.

In the Sen laboratory, genetic profiling of the 20q and 12p amplicons in four well characterized pancreatic cancer cell lines (BxPC-3, Capan-2, MIA PaCa-2, PANC-1) utilizing Agilent CGH and Expression microarray platforms has also been accomplished. The analyses employ Agilent CGH Analytics and Feature Extraction softwares. For fine mapping the amplicon boundaries along the length of each chromosome additional statistical analysis with the Circular Binary Segmentation (CBS) method is being performed. This analysis tests each defined genomic interval and selects those with liklihood ratio statistics beyond a user specified threshold based on significance level. It was proposed that utilizing the approaches described, a list of candidate biomarkers located on the common minimal amplicon intervals is being generated which will then be taken forward for validation on a test set of tumor samples.

Additionally, Dr. Marsha Frazier's laboratory has examined associations between single nucleotide polymorphisms (SNPs) in 167 patients with pancreatic cancer. SNPs in the Aurora Kinase A gene predicted early onset pancreatic cancer and in combination with p16 polymorphism, increased the risk of pancreatic cancer in a multiplicative manner. Patients with mutant genotypes for both genes had an approximately 3-fold increased age-associated risk for diagnosis of pancreatic cancer compared with wild-type genotypes.

The overall goal of this BDL is to.develop a panel of biomarkers for the early detection of pancreatic cancer utilizing locus-specific DNA based fluorescent in situ hybridization (FISH) and polymerase chain reaction (PCR) assays, protein specific immunochemical detection assays, as well as SNPs that predict early onset, methylation assays and assays for microsatelilite instability.

Diagnosis of Breast Cancer Based on DNA Methylation Profile

Anatoliy A. Melnikov[a], Denise M. Scholtens[a,b], Elizabeth L. Wiley[a,c], Seema A. Khan[a,d] and Victor V. Levenson[a,d]

[a]*Robert H. Lurie Comprehensive Cancer Center, Northwestern University, Chicago, IL, USA*
[b]*Department of Preventive Medicine, Northwestern University, Chicago, IL, USA*
[c]*Department of Pathology, Northwestern University, Chicago, IL, USA*
[d]*Department of Surgery, Feinberg School of Medicine, Northwestern University, Chicago, IL, USA*

To evaluate DNA methylation profiling for clinical diagnosis of breast cancer we compared DNA methylation in 56 promoters of cancer-related genes using 110 surgical specimens of breast cancer and 40 normal breast tissues. Breast cancer specimens represented different stages of cancer development, from atypical ductal hyperplasia (ADH) to ductal carcinoma *in situ* (DCIS) and invasive cancer. To approximate potential clinical application of the assay we used tumor-containing sections of paraffin-embedded formalin-fixed surgical material without tumor microdissection (for invasive cancer and DCIS) or material from core biopsies (for ADH). Analysis of DNA methylation was done using a modified methylation-sensitive restriction enzyme digestion with PCR (MSRE-PCR, Melnikov et al., 2005) technique with signal detection via competitive hybridization to a custom-made microarray (microarray-mediated methylation analysis, MMMA).

Method: genomic DNA from clinical specimens (2–4 ng) was divided into two aliquots, and one of them was digested with *Hin6I*, while another was incubated without the enzyme (control). Both digested and control DNA was used as templates for nested PCR with gene-specific primers. Aminoallyl-dUTP was added to the second PCR reaction, so the amplified fragments could be labeled with Cy5(control) or Cy3(digested) monoreactive dyes, and used for competitive hybridization with a custom-made oligonucleotide microarray. Normalized signals for each spot were used to calculate Cy5/Cy3 ratios and to construct corresponding methylated-unmethylated readout: if Cy5/Cy3 $= 1$ the fragment was considered methylated, while the ratio Cy5/Cy3 $\gg 1$ identified the unmethylated fragment. Reductive mammaplasty specimens served as normal control tissues; their methylation profiles were compared to profiles of other groups, and the most informative genes were selected using the Fisher's Exact Test ($p < 0.10$). The differentially methylated genes were used to construct a naïve Bayes classifier, and 25 rounds of 5-fold cross-validation were used to determine its sensitivity and specificity.

Results: sensitivity of the assay varied between 70% (for invasive cancer and DCIS) and 87.5% (for ADH), while specificity was between 73% (for invasive cancer) and 95% (for ADH). Both parameters are comparable with results of mammography.

Discussion: the pilot study shows that clinical diagnosis of breast cancer based on the DNA methylation profile is indeed possible. A larger set of informative fragments selected for ADH samples allowed higher sensitivity and specificity of the assay; the explanation is probably linked to higher purify of these specimens. We expect that use of biopsy material for analysis will make the assay more precise; increasing the number of analyzed fragments will most likely have the same result. Both venues are being explored.

Cancer Cell Type-Specific Transcriptomes for Biomarker Discovery

Alvin Y. Liu, Asa J. Oudes, Laura S. Walashek, Lawrence D. True, Hui Zhang, Priska D. von Haller and Larry W. Tjoelker
Institute for Systems Biology and MacroGenics, University of Washington, Seattle, WA, USA

Introduction and objectives: Cell type-specific transcriptomes are obtained by sorting of cell populations from tissue for gene array analysis. Compared to transcriptomes of tissue, cell transcriptomes are superior for the identification of differentially expressed genes, for example, in cancer. A comparison between the transcriptome of cancer cells in primary tumors and that of luminal cells, the normal counterpart of cancer, could uncover potentially useful biomarkers for early cancer detection.

Methods: Immunohistochemistry was done to discover differential cluster designation (CD) cell surface antigen expression between cancer (CP) and non-cancer (NP). Cell type-specific CD molecules were then used as targets for cell sorting by MACS. Surgical tissue specimens were digested by collagenase into single cells for labeling by PE-conjugated CD antibodies. The sorted cells were processed for gene expression analysis by Affymetrix DNA chips. Bioinformatics was used to identify differentially expressed genes.

Results: CD26 was used to isolated cancer cells from primary tumors. This CD26$^+$ cancer cell transcriptome was compared to that of CD26$^+$ luminal cells. Other cell transcriptomes available for analysis include those for CD104$^+$ basal epithelial cells, CD49a$^+$ stromal fibromuscular cells, CD31$^+$ endothelial cells, CDw338$^+$ (5D3) putative prostate stem/progenitor cells, prostate cancer cell lines LNCaP, C4-2, PC3 and CL1. The cancer dataset was validated by the known expression pattern of genes in cancer *vs.* normal. The different fold expression of genes identified between cancer and normal cell types was more pronounced than that between cancer and normal tissues, many of these genes (such as those encoding tight junction molecules CLDN8 and OCLN) were not discovered in previously reported tissue studies. These cancer genes showed variable expression in the cancer cell lines. Genes that encode exported proteins are especially good biomarkers for detection in body fluids. For example, the Wnt receptor FZD8 was up-regulated in the CD26$^+$ cancer cells compared to normal cells, and a Wnt1 inducible pathway signaling protein, WISP-1, peptide, K.MCAQQLGDNCTEAAICDPHR.G, was detected in glycopeptide-capture proteomic analysis of CP.

Conclusions: Cancer cell transcriptome analysis was carried out to identify cancer-specific secreted proteins that could be utilized as disease biomarkers. Isotopically labeled synthetic peptides of these proteins can be made to quantify their levels in tissue preparation, voided urine, or blood.

DNA Repair Biomarkers for Cancer Risk Assessment and Early Detection

Tamar Paz-Elizur[a], Ziv Sevilya[a], Yael Leitner-Dagan[a], Edna Schechtman[b], Ofra Barnett-Griness[c], Ronit Almog[c], Gad Rennert[c] and Zvi Livneh[a]

[a]*Department of Biological Chemistry, The Weizmann Institute of Science, Rehovot, Israel*

[b]*Department of Industrial Engineering and Management, Ben Gurion University of the Negev, Beer Sheva, Israel*

[c]*Department of Community Medicine & Epidemiology, Carmel Medical Center and Technion Faculty of Medicine, and CHS National Israeli Cancer Control Center, Haifa, Israel*

DNA repair evolved to remove DNA damage inflicted by environmental and intracellular agents, thereby providing a key mechanism for maintaining genetic stability. Mutations in DNA repair genes cause a multitude of DNA alterations including rearrangements, breakage, and increased point mutations, and therefore it is no surprise that mutations in DNA repair genes were found to be associated with several hereditary cancer predisposition syndromes. These include hereditary non-polyposis colorectal cancer (mutations in mismatch repair genes), xeroderma pigmentosum (mutations in nucleotide excision repair genes), MYH-associated polyposis (mutations in a base excision repair gene) and more. Several studies have shown that reduced DNA repair is a risk factor also in sporadic cancers such as lung cancer, however, the scarcity of functional specific DNA repair assays that are suitable for epidemiological studies hampers the progress in this field.

Our goal is to develop a series of DNA repair biomarkers for cancer risk assessment, and apply them to large-scale screening directed towards cancer prevention in general, and lung cancer prevention in particular. Our approach is based on functional DNA repair assays, and specifically enzymatic DNA repair activities. We have previously developed an enzymatic activity assay for the repair of the oxidative DNA lesion 8-oxoguanine in extracts from human peripheral blood mononuclear cells (PBMC). Using this assay evidence was obtained to indicate that reduced activity of the enzyme OGG (8-oxoguanine DNA glycosylase), which removes 8-oxoguanine from DNA, is a risk factor in lung cancer. The role of OGG activity in head and neck cancer is currently under analysis.

Under the EDRN program we have begun to develop blood tests for several DNA repair enzymes that are involved in the repair of oxidative DNA damage. We have examined four enzymes of the base excision repair pathway, and a DNA damage-prevention enzyme in extracts prepared from PBMC. Three enzymatic activities were detected and characterized using synthetic oligonucleotide substrates with defined site-specific lesions. AP endonuclease (APE1; HAP1; APEX), acting on an abasic site, methylpurine DNA glycosylase (MPG; ANPG; AAG) acting on a $1,N^6$-ethenoadenine adduct and on hypoxanthine, and thymine DNA glycosylase (TDG), acting on a $3,N^4$-ethenocytosine adduct. Two additional activities are being addressed: the adenine DNA glycosylase MYH (hMutY), and the 8-oxodGTPase activity of MTH1. At the end of the characterization step, epidemiology-grade assays will be developed for 2–3 DNA repair enzymes, and their role in lung cancer risk will be assessed.

Biomarker-Based Telecytopathology: A New Prospective for Global Cervical Cancer Control[1]

Nenad Markovic[a], Olivera Markovic[a], David Hankins[b], Lewis Townsend[c], Gene Hill[d] and Stephen McJonathan[e]
[a]*BioSciCon, Inc, Rockville, MD, USA*
[b]*World Academy for Health and Humanities, Bethesda, MD, USA*
[c]*Contemporary Women's Health Care Associates, Bethesda, MD, USA*
[d]*Computercraft, McLean, VA, USA*
[e]*GT Vision, Hagerstown, MD, USA*

Introduction: Cytological screening and the Pap test remain the most successful cervical cancer prevention strategy. However, only 6.5% of 1.7 billion women at risk worldwide receive screening and 250,000 women die each year from a preventable disease in the 21st Century. The main reasons for this "failure" are the cost of Pap test and the lack of infrastructure and qualified personnel to perform the screening. The new WHO strategy "See & Treat" and HPV testing is less effective than the Pap test. A biomarker-based telecytopathology (e.g., MarkPap[TM] Digital), a combination of biomarker cytology, digital imaging and networking via Internet, could provide an accurate, fast, low cost and affordable cervical cancer screening for low-resource areas worldwide.

Method: We have combined the first-line MarkPap® technology products with commercially available instruments (each of them fit-for-use in this application) with user-friendly software. We are now learning how to combine all of them into an integrative device with potentials for use in mass screening of cytological specimens. At this moment, we have combined an assembly of instruments including an Image Acquisition Module (microscope with digital camera, PC with image capturing, storing and image delivering ability), an Image Transferring Module (a central server to accept images from many remote sites, make them available for review of pathologists, and to report results instantly).

Results: In a pilot study, we acquired images from existing microscopic slides (from the MarkPap Library of Slides), processed them through this multi-modular device, and compared cytological results obtainable from images with those already determined on microscopic slides. We found the system is amenable for the intended use after some software modification and method optimization. We have created and transferred images around the world with little deformation. We will confirm the system once we complete the analysis of 500 slides (all TBS categories) and compare results of pathologists' review of slides and images.

Conclusion: Current results warrant continuation of this translational research. We expect this research, when completed, to introduce a prototype of a new digital image device for mass cervical cancer screening in low-resource areas, particularly in developing countries.

[1]The development of MarkPap technology was supported in part by NIH/ SBIR Grant 2R43CA80767.

Circulating Markers for Breast Cancer Discrimination Assayed by Luminex?

Jeffrey R. Marks, Alex Lisovich, Adele Marrangoni, Lyudmila Velikokhatnaya, Brian Nolen, Matthew Winans, Francesmary Modugno and Anna Lokshin
Duke University Medical Center, Durham, NC, USA
University of Pittsburgh Medical Center, Pittsburgh, PA, USA

Introduction: Early detection of breast cancer presents special challenges for biomarker development. Mammography has a large established practice base, can detect small invasive and pre-invasive lesions, and possesses a demonstrated utility in reducing breast cancer related mortality. Further, it is a non-invasive procedure that is well tolerated and relatively inexpensive. Finally, mammography provides a location that can be sampled directly to determine whether the imaged lesion is cancer or benign. For all of these positive aspects, mammography is far from a perfect test. Sensitivity for annual screening mammography is estimated to be approximately 70% while specificity can be as low as 20%. This low specificity results in approximately one million biopsies for benign conditions each year in this country. Our EDRN project is designed to provide additional information in order to discriminate between cancer and benign conditions in women with an abnormal mammogram.

Methods: Women undergoing diagnostic biopsy at Duke University Medical Center for breast cancer between 2000-2004 were enrolled in this study. Before cytoreductive surgery, women were consented for the study and blood was obtained. Serum, plasma, and white blood cells were aliquoted and cryogenically stored. Two sets were constructed from these samples: 1) Forty-two women over the age of 55 with benign breast findings and 2) Forty-six women over the age of 55 with invasive breast cancers greater than 1.5 cm. In addition, sera from 120 healthy women were used for controls. Sera were assayed for 52 different biomarkers using the Luminex platform and reagents. The biomarkers included CA 15-3, CA-125, CEA, AFP, CA 72-4, VEGF, bFGF, IGFBPI, HGF, ErbB2, EGFR, Fas, FasL, Cyfra 21-1, MMP-2, MMP-3, tPAI, sICAM, V-CAM, sE-selectin, IL-1β, IL-2, IL-4, IL-5, IL-6, IL-8, IL-10, IL-12p40, IL-13, IL-15, IL-17, IL-18, TNFα, TNFR I, TNFR II, IFNγ, GM-CSF, G-CSF, IL-2R IP-10, MCP-1, MIP-1α, MIP-1β, MIF, Eotaxin, RANTES, bHCG, kallikreins 8 and 10, mesothelin, resistin, and myeloperoxidase (MPO). We applied an adaptive density estimation (ADE) approach to the data.

Results: A 13-biomarker panel was selected using the projection pursuit technique: CA 15-3, IL-8, G-CSF, ErbB2, EGFR, Cyfra 21-1, sE-selectin, sVCAM, sICAM, MPO 31, tPAI, MIF, MMP2. When healthy women were compared with patients with breast cancer, the resulting model led to correctly classifying **84%** of the test set observations, with a sensitivity of **83%** and a specificity of **85%**. The discrimination of breast cancer from benign breast disease resulted in **68%** sensitivity at **80%** specificity.

Discussion: While these results suggest that a model to discriminate benign from malignant breast disease may be achievable with a limited number of analytes, the predictive accuracy of these models is currently insufficient to reduce the number of biopsies after an abnormal mammogram. Additional assays are currently being performed on larger sample sets. The results from this ongoing work will be presented.

Hypermethylation of the MAL Gene Promoter in Breast Cancer

Jeffrey R. Marks, Hisani Horne, Susan Murphy and Paula Lee
Duke University Medical Center, Durham, NC, USA

Introduction: We have performed several types of searches to identify novel genes that are epigenetically altered in breast and ovarian cancer. From these studies, we discovered that the CpG island associated with the MAL gene (also called T-cell differentiation protein, Hs.80395) is hypermethylated in the majority of breast cancer cell lines and primary breast cancer specimens.

Methods: Initial screening was performed via gene expression array analysis of primary ovarian and breast cancers and breast cancer cell lines treated with the demethylating agent, 5-aza-deoxycytidine (AzaC). Candidate genes were analyzed by bisulfite sequencing. Reactivation of transcription in cell culture systems was measured by Northern blotting and quantitative RT-PCR.

Results: The Mal gene, located on 2q13, was found to be the most differentially expressed gene when comparing ovarian cancer patients with good versus poor prognosis (Berchuck et al., Clin. Can. Res., 2005). By analyzing a portion of the CpG island that spans the transcriptional start site, we found that ovarian cancers had a very low frequency of hypermethylation in this region, however breast cancers were commonly methylated. By sequence analysis, we identified a region that is hypermethylated in the majority of breast cancers (30/37) and breast cancer cell lines but shows no evidence of methylation in a series of normal mammary epithelial cultures and normal lymphocytes. In addition, we demonstrate that transcription of this gene can be reactivated by 5AzaC (but not trychostatin A) in most cell lines with hypermethylation.

Discussion: The MAL gene appears to function in apical transport in polarized epithelial cells within lipid rafts. Decreased expression of MAL has been associated with cancer of the esophagus and in vitro studies suggest that it may function as a tumor suppressor gene. Our data indicate that it may well be a tumor suppressor gene in breast cancer as well given the frequency with which it is hypermethylated in the disease. We have developed a quantitative method for assessing the methylation status and are currently applying it to patient plasma.

A Suite of Assays to Detect Phosphorylated Receptor Tyrosine Kinases Associated with Neoplasia

Anu Mathew, Timothy S. Schaefer, Jane Zhang, Sean Higgins, Laura K. Schaefer, Robert M. Umek and Jacob N. Wohlstadter
Meso Scale Discovery, Gaithersburg, MD, USA

Reversible tyrosine phosphorylation is a critical process in the transduction of signals from the cell surface to the nucleus resulting in global changes in gene expression. A common hallmark of most neoplasia is the inappropriate expression or activation of cell surface proteins possessing inherent tyrosine kinase activity. These membrane spanning receptor tyrosine kinases (RTKs) phosphorylate themselves on tyrosine residues located on the cytoplasmic portion of the protein that serve as docking sites for adapter proteins. The resulting multiprotein complexes form the framework for numerous signaling pathways involved in proliferation, differentiation, angiogenesis and cell survival. Here we describe a suite of individual and multiplex assays designed to assess the level of phosphorylation of EGFR, ErbB2, VEGFR-2, PDGFR-β and c-Kit in cellular lysates which can serve as a surrogate for disease state. The assays are facile, sensitive and can be performed more rapidly than immunoblots and ELISAs and require considerably less material.

Inactivation and Restoration of Transforming Growth Factor-Beta Signaling Modulated Hepatocellular Carcinogenesis in Hepatocellular Cancer Cell Lines and $elf^{+/-}$ Tissues

K. Kitisin, N. Ganesan, E.A. Volpe, S.S. Kim, V. Katuri, Y. Tang, B. Mishra, L. Johnson, K. Shetty and L. Mishra
Georgetown University, Washington, DC, USA

Hepatocellular cancer (HCC) is the fifth most common solid malignancy worldwide and is increasing in the United States. Nearly 500,000 cases of HCC are diagnosed each year, prognosis remaining extremely poor. Recent studies in human HCCs reveal the emergence of transforming growth factor-beta (TGF-beta) as a key signaling pathway in suppressing these cancers through Smad proteins and adaptor proteins such as the embryonic liver fodrin (ELF). TGF-beta can induce antiproliferative gene responses by inhibiting cellular progression in G1 phase. Arrested cells in the G1 phase display downregulation in expression of Cdk2, Cdk4, cyclin D1, cyclin D2, cyclin D3 and cyclin A. Escape from this response is a hallmark of many cancer cells. Importantly, our lab has demonstrated that as many as 35% of $elf^{+/-}$ mice (7/20) developed HCC spontaneously and showed additional phenotypic changes such as increased centrilobular steatosis and high grade dysplasia.

Aims: 1. To determine whether ELF and TGF-beta signaling proteins are inactivated in human HCC cell lines 2. To analyze the changes in cell cycle regulation in wild type mouse embryonic fibroblasts (MEF) and $elf^{-/-}$ MEF cell lines. 3. To investigate whether restoration of ELF can reverse the aberration of cell cycle regulation.

Methods and Results: 1. Expression of ELF and other proteins involved in the TGF-beta signaling pathway, particularly Smad2, Smad4 and TGF-beta receptor II (TBRII), were examined in human HCC cell lines SNU-182, SNU-398, SNU-449, and SNU-475. ELF expression was lost in one human HCC cell line (SNU-398), and decreased in SNU-182 and SNU-475. Smad 2 expression was lost in all five HCC cell lines. TBRII expression was lost in three cell lines (SNU-398, SNU-182, and SNU-475). 2. Further analysis of the role of ELF in human HCC confirms markedly reduced nuclear expression of ELF in 9 out of 10 human HCC samples by immunohistochemistry. 3. Immortalized $elf^{-/-}$ MEF cell lines showed a marked increase in Cdk4 level by 3-4 times. 4. Immunohistochemical labeling of $elf^{+/-}$ HCC tissue revealed markedly increased cyclin D1. 5. Restoration of ELF protein in human HCC cell line, SNU-182, results in a decrease in cyclin D1 protein expression via Western blot analysis.

Conclusions: Diminished or absent ELF expression in mouse and human HCC as well as cell cycle deregulation are due to disruption of TGF-beta signaling. Loss of ELF can serve as a primary event in progression towards a fully transformed phenotype. Exploration of the mechanisms behind inactivation of the TGF-beta signaling pathway and its restoration holds promise for new diagnostic and therapeutic approaches in human hepatocellular cancer.

TGF-Beta/Smads Regulate a Wide Variety of Biological Responses through Transcriptional Regulation of Target Genes

V. Katuri, Y. Tang, B. Marshall, A. Rashid, W. Jogunoori, E.A. Volpe, A.N. Sidawy, S. Evans, J. Blay, G.I. Gallicano, Reddy E. Premkumar, L. Mishra and B. Mishra
Department of Surgical Sciences, Medicine Laboratory of Developmental Molecular Biology, , Lombardi Cancer Center, Georgetown University, Washington, DC, USA

TGF-beta/Smads regulate a wide variety of biological responses through transcriptional regulation of target genes. ELF, a beta-spectrin, plays a key role in the transmission of TGF-beta-mediated transcriptional response through Smads. ELF was originally identified as a key protein involved in endodermal stem/progenitor cells committed to foregut lineage. Also, as a major dynamic adaptor and scaffolding protein, ELF is important for the generation of functionally distinct membranes, protein sorting and the development of polarized differentiated epithelial cells. Disruption of elf results in the loss of Smad3/Smad4 activation and, therefore, a disruption of the TGF-beta pathway. These observations led us to pursue the function of ELF in gastric (GI) epithelial cell-cell adhesion and tumor suppression. Here, we show a significant loss of ELF and reduced Smad4 expression in human gastric cancer tissue samples. Also, of the six human gastric cancer cell lines examined, three show deficient ELF expression. Furthermore, we demonstrate the rescue of E-cadherin-dependent homophilic cell-cell adhesion by ectopic expression of full-length elf. Our results suggest that ELF has an essential role in tumor suppression in GI cancers, and could represent a strong marker for the detection and prognosis of gastric cancers.

Transforming Growth Factor-Beta Suppresses Non-metastatic Colon Cancer Through Smad4 and Adaptor Protein ELF at an Early Stage of Tumorigenesis

Y. Tang, V. Katuri, R. Srinivasan, F. Fogt, R. Redman, G. Anand, A. Said, T. Fishbein, M. Zasloff, E.P. Reddy, B. Mishra and L. Mishra
Laboratory of GI Developmental Biology, Department of Surgery, Lombardi Cancer Center, Georgetown University, Washington, DC, USA

Although transforming growth factor-beta (TGF-beta) is both a suppressor and promoter of tumorigenesis, its contribution to early tumor suppression and staging remains largely unknown. In search of the mechanism of early tumor suppression, we identified the adaptor protein ELF, a beta-spectrin from stem/progenitor cells committed to foregut lineage. ELF activates and modulates Smad4 activation of TGF-beta to confer cell polarity, to maintain cell architecture, and to inhibit epithelial-to-mesenchymal transition. Analysis of development of colon cancer in (adult) elf+/−/Smad4+/−, elf+/−, Smad4+/−, and gut epithelial cells from elf−/− mutant mouse embryos pinpoints the defect to hyperplasia/adenoma transition. Further analysis of the role of ELF in human colorectal cancer confirms reduced expression of ELF in Dukes' B1 stage tissues ($P < 0.05$) and of Smad4 in advanced colon cancers ($P < 0.05$). This study indicates that by modulating Smad 4, ELF has a key role in TGF-beta signaling in the suppression of early colon cancer. Elf as well as Smad4 could play a key role in detection of B2 cancers and thus present as a prognostic indicator.

RTPCR Detection of Cancer Cells in Blood Based on Presence of a tNOX Splice Variant mRNA

D. James Morre, Xiaoyu Tang, Dorothy M. Morre, Kenneth L. Pennington, Heather Hignite, Helen Orvis and Douglas J. Schwartzentruber
Department of Medicinal Chemistry and Molecular Pharmacology, Purdue University, West Lafayette, IN, USA
NOX Technologies, Inc., West Lafayette, IN, USA
Department of Foods and Nutrition, Purdue University, West Lafayette, IN, USA
Center for Cancer Care, Goshen, IN, USA

A novel hydroquinone and NADH oxidase with protein disulfide-thiol interchange activity (designated tNOX), is associated exclusively with the outer leaflet of the plasma membrane at the surface of cancer cells. Also present in sera of cancer patients, it is absent from the surface of non-cancer cells and from sera from healthy individuals. Nevertheless, tNOX mRNA has approximately the same abundance in both normal and cancer cells. Our research demonstrates alternative splicing as the basis for the cancer specificity of tNOX expression at the cell surface.

We have developed probes to detect by RTPCR a 150 bp product indicative of tNOX splice variant mRNA in the blood of cancer patients. Venous blood was collected into 7 ml vacutainers containing potassium EDTA. The specimens were snap frozen and stored at $-80°$ C until RNA extraction. Total RNA from whole peripheral blood was extracted using a Fast Lane Cell cDNA kit (Qiagen). Purity and amounts of total RNA were assessed by electrophoresis in Tris-Acetate-EDTA buffer on 1% agarose gels, with the DNA bands visualized by ethidium bromide staining. We evaluated 40 patients with histologic diagnosis of breast, lung, or ovarian cancer and 20 healthy volunteers. The specificity and sensitivity of the procedure was established initially using human cancer cell lines in culture (HeLa cervical carcinoma, BT-20 mammary carcinoma, MCF-10 mammary non-cancer.) Splice variant-specific tNOX primers were designed according to published sequence information (Available from GenBank under Accession No. AF 207881). Each RT-PCR run included a positive control (tNOX-positive cell line or blood donor) and blood from a negative donor. Under the assay conditions developed, 70% of patients with cancer were positive for tNOX slice variant mRNA. Samples from individuals free of disease or with disorders other than cancer were negative. Our expectation is that this assay will provide a tool for detecting cancer cells in the circulation. Larger cohorts will be required in future studies to define the utility of this technology to detect splice variant-tNOX mRNA in blood borne cells in cancer management.

tNOX a Circulating Pancancer Marker Potentially Indicative of Cancer Presence

D. James Morre
NOX Technologies/Purdue University, West Lafayette, IN, USA

We are developing technology based on the discovery from our laboratories of a family of cell surface oxidases (hydroquinone or NADH as substrates) with protein disulfide- thiol interchange activity designated as ECTO (for external cell surface)-NOX (for <u>N</u>ADH <u>ox</u>idase) proteins. One member of the ECTO-NOX family, tNOX (for tumor-associated NOX), is uniquely drug inhibited and cancer specific. As is characteristic of ectoproteins in general, ECTO-NOX proteins are shed from the cell surface and accumulate in the circulation based on enzymatic assays of drug- (antitumor sulfonylurea- or capsaicin-) inhibited oxidation of NADH by samples of patient sera. The molecular basis for the cancer specificity of tNOX is due to a cancer-specific exon-4 minus splice variant yielding a mRNA capable of initiation at a down-stream methonine. The protein product of the exon-4 minus truncation is then processed to a mature 34 kD tNOX form and delivered to the cell surface. tNOX has been cloned [1] and overexpressed in bacteria (as a source of recombinant protein) and in COS cells and non-cancer human mammary MCF-10A cells as a means of target validation.

tNOX overexpression in both cultured non-cancer cells and in mice leads to more rapid growth (larger cells and increased body weight) and a drug response not seen prior to transfection. Transfected non-cancer MCF-10A cells acquire cancer-like invasive ability (proliferation in Matrigel) [2]. Treatment with antisense restores the normal growth phenotype to HeLa cells (loss of ability to form colonies on soft agar). A protocol developed to utilize RT-PCR for the detection of occult metastases in blood samples of cancer patients is being evaluated for potential prognostic value in the detection of disseminated disease. The focused objective of the work proposed is to generate one or more additional tNOX specific reagents (antisera and/or RT-PCR olignouncleotide probes) and/or protocols suitable for distribution to outside laboratories and investigators and as a first step toward proof-of-concept for the potential utility of the tNOX target in cancer detection and control.

References

[1] P.-J. Chueh, C. Kim, N.M. cho, D.M. Morre and D.J. Morre, Molecular cloning and characterization of a tumor-associated, growth-related, and time-keeping hydroquinone (NADH) oxidase (tNOX) of the HeLa cell surface, *Biochemistry* **41** (2002), 3732–3741.

[2] P.-J. Chueh, L.-Y. Wu, D.M. Morre and D.J. Morre, tNOX is both necessary and sufficient as a cellular target for the anticancer actions of capsaicin and the green tea catechin(-)-epigallocatechin-3-gallate, *BioFactors* **20** (2004), 249–263.

Deletions of the *TSPY* Gene Cluster in Prostate Cancer[1]

S. Vijayakumar, D.C. Hall, X.T. Reveles, D.A. Troyer, I.M. Thompson, D.K. Garcia, R.H. Xiang, R.J. Leach, T.L. Johnson-Pais and S.L. Naylor
The University of Texas Health Science Center, San Antonio, TX, USA

We have previously shown that introduction of the human Y chromosome by microcell hybridization suppresses the *in vivo* tumorigenicity of the prostate cancer cell line, PC-3. To determine whether we could observe deletions of the Y chromosome in prostate tumors, we developed a high-density bacterial artificial chromosome (BAC) microarray containing 178 BAC clones from the human Y chromosome. Spectral Genomics printed this array. Prostate cancer samples and cell lines were analyzed by array comparative genomic hybridization (aCGH). Dissected prostate tumor samples had deletion at Yp11.2 containing the *TSPY* tandem gene array in 16 out of 36 primary prostate tumors (44.4%). Moreover, PC-3 hybrids with an intact Yp11.2 did not grow tumors in nude mice, while PC-3 hybrids with a deletion at Yp11.2 grew tumors in nude mice. The deletion was verified by real time PCR and reduced expression of TSPY was noted by RT PCR. T*SPY* copy number was determined in the blood samples from men with and with out prostate cancer. There was a correlation with the incidence of prostate cancer and a low copy number of TSPY.

[1]Supported by EDRN, the Department of Defense, and the San Antonio Cancer Institute.

Obesity, Adipokines, and Prostate Cancer in a Prospective Population-Based Study

Jacques Baillargeon[a,b], Elizabeth A. Platz[c], David P. Rose[a], Brad H. Pollock[a,b,d], Donna Pauler Ankerst[e], Steven Haffner[d], Betsy Higgins[f], Anna Lokshin[g], Dean Troyer[h], Javier Hernandez[i], Steve Lynch[j] and Ian M. Thompson[f]
[a]*Center for Epidemiology and Biostatistics, University of Texas Health Science Center, San Antonio, TX, USA*
[b]*Department of Pediatrics, University of Texas Health Science Center, San Antonio, TX, USA*
[c]*Department of Epidemiology, Johns Hopkins Bloomberg School of Public Health, Baltimore, MD, USA*
[d]*Department of Medicine, University of Texas Health Science Center, San Antonio, TX, USA*
[e]*Institute for Medical Informatics, Biometry and Epidemiology, University of Munich, Germany*
[f]*Department of Urology, University of Texas Health Science Center, San Antonio, TX, USA*
[g]*University of Pittsburgh Cancer Center, Pittsburgh, PA, USA*
[h]*Department of Pathology, University of Texas Health Science Center, San Antonio, TX, USA*
[i]*Brooke Army Medical Center, San Antonio, TX, USA*
[j]*Wilford Hall Medical Center, San Antonio, TX, USA*

Objective: The purpose of this investigation was to examine the association of obesity and the adipokines leptin, adiponectin, and interleukin-6 (IL-6) with prostate cancer risk and aggressiveness.

Methods: 125 incident prostate cancer cases and 125 age-matched controls were sampled from among participants in the original San Antonio Center for Biomarkers of Risk of Prostate Cancer (SABOR) cohort study. The odds ratios (OR) of prostate cancer and high-grade disease (Gleason sum $\geqslant 7$) associated with the World Health Organization categories of body mass index (BMI, kg/m^2) and with tertiles of serum concentrations of adiponectin, leptin, and IL-6 were estimated using multivariable conditional logistic regression models.

Results: BMI was not associated with either incident prostate cancer (obese vs. normal, OR = 0.75, 95% CI 0.38–1.48, P trend = 0.27) or high-grade disease (OR = 1.17, 95% CI, 0.39–3.52, P trend = 0.62). Moreover, none of the three adipokines was statistically significant associated with prostate cancer risk or high-grade disease, respectively: leptin (highest vs. lowest tertile, OR = 0.77, 95% CI 0.28–1.37, P trend = 0.57; 1.20, 95% CI 0.48–3.01, P trend = 0.85); adiponectin

(OR $= 0.87$, 95% CI 0.46–1.65, P trend $= 0.24$; OR $= 1.93$, 95% CI 0.74–5.10, P trend $= 0.85$); IL-6 (OR $= 0.84$, 95% CI 0.46–1.53, P trend $= 0.98$; OR $= 0.84$, 95% CI 0.30–2.33 P trend $= 0.17$).

Conclusions: Findings from this nested case-control study of men routinely screened for prostate cancer and who had a high prevalence of overweight and obesity do not provide evidence to support that obesity or factors elaborated by fat cells strongly influence prostate cancer risk or aggressiveness.

Recurrent Homozygous Deletion on Chromosome 18q22.3 in Prostate Cancer

Devon C. Hall, Xavier T. Reveles, Sapna Vijayakumar, Dean A. Troyer, Ian M. Thompson, Susan L. Naylor, Teresa L. Johnson-Pais and Robin J. Leach
The University of Texas Health Science Center at San Antonio, TX, USA

Prostate cancer has a major genetic component. Chromosomal deletions, as well as amplification, are a common finding in these tumors. The majority of the chromosome losses involve the loss of a single copy of a gene and/or regions. Here we report a homozygous deletion on chromosome 18q22.3 which was present in the majority (11/19) of prostate tumors evaluated by a high resolution genomic array developed for the distal end of chromosome 18q. Fluorescence in situ hybridization (FISH) analysis of paraffin-embedded tumor samples verified the deletion in 100% of the original prostate samples analyzed (5/5) using the bacterial artificial clone from the array. Further characterization of tumors on tissue arrays demonstrated that the homozygous deletion was present in a subset of breast tumors but absent in 10 other tumors types including colorectal, esophageal, stomach, renal, lung, bladder, thyroid, liver, ovary and pancreas. Using tyramide signal amplification (TSA) FISH analysis, the region of loss has been narrowed to less than 150 kb, contained within a single bacterial artificial chromosome. TSA FISH also demonstrated that the tumors had different breakpoints. This supports our hypothesis that the region is not lost because of repetitive elements associated with an unstable phenotype as seen in many cancers. This region does not appear to contain any genes that are expressed in the prostate, however only two known genes have currently been identified. Furthermore, it does contain putative estrogen response elements and the loss is limited to cancer with are hormonally regulated. Therefore, this region could harbor a cryptic tumor suppressor gene and/or regulatory sequence that has yet to be identified.

The VEGF +405 CC Polymorphism Is Associated with Prostate Cancers of Poor Prognosis

Edith Canby-Hagino, Dawn Garcia, Ian Thompson, Dean Troyer, Jacques Baillargeon, Timothy Brand, Robin Leach and Susan Naylor
The University of Texas Health Science Center at San Antonio, TX, USA

Introduction and objectives: Vascular endothelial growth factor (VEGF) supports growth and metastasis of malignant neoplasms, including prostate cancer. A single nucleotide polymorphism (SNP) of the VEGF gene positioned at +405 is associated with increased production of VEGF protein and neovascularity in nonmalignant conditions. We examined this SNP in a case-control study to determine ethnic distribution of allelic frequency, prostate cancer risk and prognosis associated with this variant.

Materials and methods: A total of 1570 consecutively enrolled volunteers enrolled in the San Antonio Center of Biomarkers of Risk for Prostate Cancer (SABOR) prospective cohort study were genotyped using Taqman allelic discrimination assays to determine allelic frequency of the VEGF +405 C/G SNP. Case-control analysis was performed on 646 cases and 1068 controls to assess the association between this SNP and prostate cancer risk and prognosis. Controls were limited to male participants in SABOR who were older than 40 years with a normal prostate examination, a serum PSA of $\leqslant 2.5$ ng/ml, and no diagnosis of prostate cancer. Cases included individuals with incident prostate cancer diagnosed through the SABOR program as well as individuals with a history of prostate cancer accrued from the greater San Antonio area.

Results: Allelic frequency of the VEGF +405 SNP varied significantly among different ethnic groups. In the total study population, a diagnosis of prostate cancer was not significantly associated with increased odds for any VEGF +405 genotype. However, logistic regression analysis adjusted for age and stratified by ethnicity demonstrated significant association between the CC genotype at this locus and prostate cancers of poor prognosis, as determined by Gleason score and stage. The CC genotype was associated with an increased risk for prostate cancer with a Gleason grade of 7 or higher for all ethnicities, with an odds ratio (OR) of 1.97 (95% CI 1.120–3.479). The CC genotype was most strongly associated with this higher Gleason score in Hispanics, with an OR of 3.31 (95% CI 1.022–10.701). In addition, for the entire population, the CC genotype was associated with prostate cancers of bad outcome, as determined by Gleason score of 8 or higher or stage T3b or higher, with an OR of 2.42 (95% CI 1.286–4.567). This association was also significant for the subgroup of non-Hispanic Caucasians (OR 2.25, 95% CI 1.043–4.876).

Conclusions: Allelic frequency of the VEGF +405 C/G SNP varies significantly across ethnicity, and the CC genotype at VEGF +405 is associated with prostate cancers of poor prognosis, as determined by Gleason score and stage.

Variants of Semaphorin 3F Are Associated with Prostate Cancer Prognosis

Timothy C. Brand, Edith D. Canby-Hagino, Dawn Garcia, Jacques Baillargeon, Dean A. Troyer, Ian M. Thompson, Robin J. Leach and Susan L. Naylor
The University of Texas Health Science Center at San Antonio, San Antonio, TX, USA

Introduction and objectives: Semaphorin 3F (SEMA3F) on chromosome 3 has been shown to suppress tumor formation *in vivo* and *in vitro*. We examined two single nucleotide polymorphisms in this gene in a case-control study to determine CaP risk and prognosis associated with variants of SEMA3F. The loci of interest were SEMA3F rs2073726 and SEMA3F rs13067082.

Materials and methods: For SEMA3F rs2073726, 684 cases and 1101 controls were genotyped, and for SEMA3F rs13067082, 635 cases and 834 controls were genotyped. Controls were limited to male participants in the San Antonio Center of Biomarkers of Risk for Prostate Cancer (SABOR) prospective cohort study who were older than 40 years with a normal prostate examination and a prostate specific antigen $\leqslant$ 2.5 ng/ml, and no diagnosis of prostate cancer. Cases included individuals with incident prostate cancer diagnosed through the SABOR program as well as individuals with a history of prostate cancer accrued from the greater San Antonio area.

Results: In the total study population, a diagnosis of prostate cancer was not significantly associated with increased odds for either SEMA3F polymorphism, but polymorphisms at these loci were associated with cancers of poor prognosis, as determined by Gleason score and stage. The presence of any A allele at SEMA3F rs2073726 was associated with an increased risk for prostate cancer with a Gleason grade of 7 or higher in non-Hispanic Caucasians, with an odds ratio (OR) of 2.97 (95% CI 1.466–6.034) for the AA genotype, and OR of 2.47 (95% CI 1.289–4.742) for the AT genotype. In addition, the AG genotype at SEMA3F rs13067082 was associated with cancers with Gleason score 7 or higher with an OR of 6.56 (95% CI 1.069–40.292) in the African-American group.

Conclusions: Polymorphisms in SEMA3F at rs2073726 and rs13067082 are associated with prostate cancers of worse prognosis.

The Effect of Finasteride on the Sensitivity of PSA for Detecting Prostate Cancer

Ian M. Thompson[a], Chen Chi[b], Donna Pauler Ankerst[c], Phyllis J. Goodman[b], Catherine M. Tangen[b], Scott M. Lippman[d], M. Scott Lucia[e], Howard L. Parnes[f], Charles A. Coltman, Jr.[g] and Susan L. Naylor[h]
[a]*Department of Urology, University of Texas HSC, San Antonio, TX, USA*
[b]*Fred Hutchinson Cancer Research Center, Seattle, WA, USA*
[c]*Institute for Medical Informatics, Biometry and Epidemiology, University of Munich, Germany*
[d]*Department of Clinical Cancer Prevention, The University of Texas M. D. Anderson Cancer Center, Houston, TX, USA*
[e]*Department of Pathology, University of Colorado HSC, Denver, CO, USA*
[f]*Division of Cancer Prevention, National Cancer Institute, Bethesda, MD, USA*
[g]*The Southwest Oncology Group, San Antonio, TX, USA*
[h]*The University of Texas Health Science Center at San Antonio, TX, USA*

Background: The operating characteristics of prostate-specific antigen (PSA) are better for detecting higher than lower grade prostate cancer (PCA). We examined the impact of the 5??-reductase inhibitor finasteride on the sensitivity and area underneath the receiver operating characteristic curve (AUC) of PSA in the Prostate Cancer Prevention Trial (PCPT).

Methods: Study participants included men in the placebo and finasteride groups of the PCPT who had a prostate biopsy and PSA within one year of biopsy. The sensitivity and AUC for PSA was compared between finasteride and placebo for PCA versus no PCA, Gleason grade $\geqslant 7$ versus Gleason $\leqslant 6$ or no PCA, and Gleason $\geqslant 8$ versus Gleason $\leqslant 7$ or no PCA.

Results: Of 5,112 men in the placebo group, 1,111 had PCA. Tumor grade was available in 1,100: 240 had Gleason $\geqslant 7$ and 55 had Gleason $\geqslant 8$. Of 4,579 men in the finasteride group, 695 had PCA, graded in 686: 264 had Gleason $\geqslant 7$ and 81 had Gleason $\geqslant 8$. The AUC was greater for finasteride than placebo: PCA versus no PCA: 0.757 (finasteride) versus 0.681 (placebo) ($p < 0.001$); Gleason $\geqslant 7$: 0.838 versus 0.781 ($p = 0.003$); Gleason $\geqslant 8$: 0.886 versus 0.824 ($p = 0.071$). The sensitivity of PSA was higher on finasteride than placebo at all PSA cut-offs matched by specificity.

Conclusions: PSA had significantly better sensitivity for PCA detection in the finasteride group of the PCPT, a bias that would be expected to contribute to higher numbers of high-grade PCA in this study group.

Assessing Prostate Cancer Risk: Results from the Prostate Cancer Prevention Trial

Susan L. Naylor, Ian M. Thompson, Chen Chi, Phyllis J. Goodman, Catherine M. Tangen, P.H., M. Scott Lucia, Ziding Feng, Howard L. Parnes and Charles A. Coltman, Jr.
The University of Texas Health Science Center at San Antonio, TX, USA
The Fred Hutchinson Cancer Research Center, Seattle, WA, USA
University of Colorado, Denver, CO, USA
The Division of Cancer Prevention, National Cancer Institute, Bethesda, MD, USA
Southwest Oncology Group, San Antonio, TX, USA

Background: Prostate-specific antigen (PSA) testing is the primary screening test for prostate cancer in the United States. Methods to integrate other factors associated with the risk of prostate cancer into clinical decision-making are needed. We used prostate biopsy data from men who participated in the Prostate Cancer Prevention Trial (PCPT) to evaluate the independent contributions of PSA level and other risk factors for the prediction of prostate cancer.

Methods: We included 5519 men from the placebo group of the PCPT who underwent prostate biopsy, had at least one PSA measurement and a digital rectal examination (DRE) performed during the year before the end-of-study biopsy, and had at least two PSA measurements performed during the 3 years prior to prostate biopsy. Logistic regression was used to model the risk of prostate cancer associated with age at biopsy, race, family history of prostate cancer, PSA level, PSA velocity, DRE result, and previous prostate biopsy. All statistical tests were two-sided.

Results: A total of 1211 (21.9%) men were diagnosed with prostate cancer. Variables that predicted prostate cancer included higher PSA level, positive family history of prostate cancer, abnormal DRE result, while a previous negative prostate biopsy reduced the risk. Neither age at biopsy nor PSA velocity contributed independent prognostic information. Higher PSA level, abnormal DRE result, older age at biopsy, and African American race were predictive for high-grade disease (Gleason score $\geqslant 7$) while previous negative prostate biopsy reduced this risk.

Conclusions: This predictive model was developed from a large group of men who underwent prostate biopsy regardless of their PSA levels and DRE results. It allows an individualized assessment of prostate cancer risk and risk of high grade disease for men who undergo a prostate biopsy. Risk of detecting prostate cancer and high grade prostate cancer is calculated based on PSA level, race, family history of prostate cancer, DRE result, and history of previous prostate biopsy.

Heterogeneity in HPV 16 DNA Methylation Assessed by Pyrosequencing

M.S. Rajeevan, D. Swan, K. Duncan, J.R. Limor and E.R. Unger
Centers for Disease Control and Prevention, Atlanta, GA, USA

Background: Quantitation of HPV 16 DNA and E6/E7 transcripts in exfoliated cervical cells demonstrate that most HPV 16 is transcriptionally silent, most likely due to CpG methylation of the viral genome. HPV methylation could affect HPV oncogenesis, and potentially serve as a biomarker of cervical neoplasia. The purpose of this study was to use pyrosequencing to quantitatively evaluate the CpG methylation in LCR/E6 region of HPV 16.

Methods: We used cell lines with integrated HPV 16 as controls [CaSki ~ 400 copies and SiHa 1–2 copies] and piloted the result on HPV 16 positive exfoliated cervical and anal cells. DNA was bisulfite treated using the EZ DNA methylation kit. Methylated CpG sites were determined for the LCR/E6 region (nt 7000-194), and PCR and sequencing primers were designed using PSQ Assay Design Software. Of the 21 potentially methylated CpG sites in the LCR/E6 region, we studied all but 2 CpG sites in the region of unknown significance. As a result of bisulfite treatment and PCR, unmethylated cytosines [C] are converted to thymidines [T]. Pyrosequencing determines the proportion of C/T at each CpG site, and therefore the extent of methylation [0-100%]. Pyrosequencing was performed with PSQ 96MA system.

Results: In SiHa and cervical samples the CpG sites at nucleotide positions 7862, 31, 37, 43, 52 and 58 had 0% methylation whereas these sites were methylated 15%, 87%, 100, 95, 100 and 98% respectively in CaSki. HPV 16 DNA in both CaSki (30–100%) and SiHa (81–85%) were heavily methylated in CpG sites at nucleotide positions 7032, 7091, 7136 and 7145. In some cervical samples, the proportion of methylated CpG at 7694 ranged from 32–87%. Pyrosequencing reproducibly (SD $\pm$ 1.52) assessed CpG methylaiton levels in HPV 16 DNA with the detection limit of one CaSki cell in the background of 300, 000 HPV negative cells, and in one SiHA cell in the background of 3000 HPV negative cells.

Conclusion: In contrast to previous methods, pyrosequencing provides quantitative assessment of CpG methylation without cloning. HPV DNA methylation levels varied by CpG sites in CaSki, SiHa and cervical samples. Correlation of methylation with disease and viral transcript levels is planned.

Funding: Supported in part by NCI Early Detection Research Network IAA Y1-CN-5005-01.

Characterization of Telomerase-Immortalized Primary Non-Malignant and Malignant Tumor-Derived Human Prostate Epithelial Cell Cultures

Yongpeng Gu, Hongzhen Li, Jun Miki, Kee-Hong Kim, Bungo Furusato, Isabell A. Sesterhenn, Wei-Sing Chu, David G. McLeod, Charles M Ewing, Shiv Srivastava, William B. Isaacs and Johng S. Rhim
Center for Prostate Disease Research, USUHS, Bethesda, MD, USA
Armed Forces Institutes of Pathology, Washington, DC, USA
Walter Reed Army Medical Center, Washington, DC, USA
Johns Hopkins Medical Institutes, Baltimore, MD, USA

Introduction and objectives: Prostate cell lines can provide powerful model systems for the study of human prostate carcinogenesis. However, the human prostate cell lines (PC3, DU145 and LNCaP) studied most extensively by investigators were established from metastatic lesions, and it is unlikely that they accurately reflect the genetic makeup or biological behavior of primary prostate tumors. Cell lines ideal for the study of human prostate primary tumors would be those derived from spontaneously immortalized cells; unfortunately, explanted primary prostate cells survive only short-term in culture, and rarely immortalize spontaneously. Therefore, we examined whether cell lines generated through telomerase-transduced immortalization of primary human non-malignant and primary tumor prostate epithelium express aspects of the non-malignant or malignant phenotypes, and could serve as appropriate models for non-malignant or transformed human prostate epithelium.

Materials and methods: To accomplish these goals, we examined the phenotypic expression of cell cultures established through the immortalization of non-malignant (RC-165N and RC-170N) and malignant (957E, RC-58T and RC92a) primary human prostate epithelium with telomerase, the gene that prevents cellular senescence.

Results: Examinations of these cell lines for their morphologies and proliferous capacities, for their abilities to grow with or without serum, for their response to androgen stimulation, for their growth above the agar layer, and their ability to form tumors in SCID mice, suggests that they may serve as valid, useful tools for the elucidation of prostate tumorigenesis. Furthermore, the chromosome alterations observed in these immortalized cell lines expressing aspects of the malignant phenotypes imply that these cell lines accurately recapitulate the genetic composition of primary prostate tumors.

Conclusion: Telomerase – immortalized primary non-malignant and malignant derived human prostate epithelial cell line may be useful models for study of prostate cancer and for testing both chemopreventive and chemotherapeutic agents.

Prediction Models for Recurrence and Survival Following Surgery in Stage IA and IB NSCLC

David Ost and William Rom
New York University, NY, USA

Background: Whether or not the specific histologic subtype of non-small cell carcinoma (NSCLC) makes a clinically significant difference in terms of prognosis is unclear.

Hypothesis: The goal of this study was to develop a prediction model for patients undergoing surgery for stage IA, IB NSCLC using the SEER-Medicare database. Our specific hypothesis was that we can predict mortality more effectively by integrating tumor size and histologic subtype into existing models rather than relying solely on conventional TNM staging without specifying histologic subtypes.

Methods: We used the SEER tumor registry database to generate the study cohort. The inclusion criteria were: 1) primary NSCLC, 2) potentially curative primary surgery, defined as a wedge resection, segmentectomy, lobectomy, bilobectomy, or pneumonectomy, 3) surgical pathology stage IA or IB disease, and 4) lymph node dissections done at the time of surgery. Exclusion criteria were: 1) second primary tumors, 2) patients with a lung cancer other than NSCLC (such as small cell carcinoma, carcinoid tumors of the lung, lymphoma, etc.), and 3) not a potentially curative primary surgery as defined above. The primary outcome was time to death. We used the Cox proportional hazards and Kaplan-Meier methods to assess the relationship between variables and mortality. Comparison of models was done using the -2log-likelihood method.

Results: From 1998–2000, 8,563 patients were included. Multivariate Cox analysis demonstrated that size (HR 1.315 (95% CI 1.266–1.366), $p < 0.0001$) and adenocarcinoma histology (HR 1.088 (95% CI 1.013–1.170), $p = 0.0212$) were associated with associated with all-cause mortality. The proportional hazard due to larger tumors was attenuated somewhat with time (Interaction size x time in months HR 0.997 (95% CI 0.996–0.998), $p < 0.0001$). Multivariate Cox analysis also demonstrated that size (HR 1.465 (95% CI 1.381–1.554), $p < 0.0001$; interaction size x time in months HR 0.995 (95% CI 0.994–0.997) was also associated with death due to cancer. The proportional hazard of death due to cancer for those with adenocarcinoma also increased with time from surgery (interaction adenocarcinoma histology × time in months HR 1.008 (95% CI 1.005–1.012), $p < 0.0001$), indicating that late recurrences of adenocarcinoma were more common than with other forms of NSCLC and were driving lung cancer mortality. Compared to the standard TNM classification model, precisely specifying the size of the tumor in centimeters rather than dichotomizing size ($p < 0.0001$) and then adding tumor histology ($p = 0.021$) improved the performance of the model above and beyond that of the standard TNM system. The greatest discordance between the complete model and the standard TNM prediction were in those patients with adenocarcinomas 2–3 cm in size (TNM overestimates survival probability) and those with squamous cell carcinoma 3–4 cm in size (TNM underestimates survival).

Conclusions: We need to reevaluate our approach to the staging of NSCLC. More precise staging, taking into account size and histology, offers significant benefits. This is clinically important since improved prediction is central to making decisions on the use of adjuvant chemotherapy.

Esophageal Adenocarcinoma and Barrett's Esophagus Clinical Data, Blood and Tissue Bank

Yvonne Romero
Mayo Clinic, USA

Background: Gastroesophageal reflux is a risk factor for Barrett's esophagus (BE) and adenocarcinoma (ACA) of the esophagus, but not squamous cell carcinoma (SCCA) of the esophagus. BE is diagnosed upon the endoscopic recognition of an abnormal esophageal lining with biopsy confirmation of specialized intestinal metaplastic glands. Although BE is a premalignant disease, few BE patients will develop ACA (0.5%/yr). Due to limitations in length of follow-up and sample size it has been difficult for any single center to identify genetic pathways important in the neoplastic transformation from BE to ACA or novel biomarkers of risk, early detection or treatment response.

Aim: To create the necessary infrastructure to help address important questions with enough power to achieve meaningful results our multidisciplinary team developed a resource of blood, fixed- and fresh-frozen tissue, questionnaires, and linked clinical and pathologic data prospectively collected in a serial fashion over time.

Methods: The Esophageal Adenocarcinoma and Barrett's Esophagus (EABE) Registry began enrollment on September 10, 2001. Patients with: 1) Long segment BE (LSBE) alone; 2) LSBE with ACA; 3)

ACA alone; or 4) SCCA, as controls, are invited to participate. If willing, written informed consent is obtained. Participants complete baseline and annual validated quality of life and symptom questionnaires. Blood is collected once. Tissue (frozen and formalin-fixed) is collected at every clinically indicated endoscopic or surgical procedure.

Results: As of January 29th, 2006, 2226 patients have met entry criteria of whom 563 declined to participate, 120 died before consent, 69 were excluded, and 231 are being processed. 1243 have given consent (696 LSBE alone, 200 ACA alone, 213 LSBE with ACA, and 99 SCCA). Blood and tissue have been collected at least once from 879 and 491unique participants.

Conclusions: Identification and validation of biomarkers requires the resources of a large bank of meticulously captured and well-characterized fresh-frozen tissue, blood, demographic, symptom and risk factor data, captured serially over time. The EABE Registry provides this unique resource to help scientists and clinicians address important questions with sufficient power to yield meaningful results. We are in the planing stages of extending this resource to other institutions committed to research in BE and ACA.

Identifying Molecular Signatures of Indolent and Aggressive Prostate Cancer

Mark A. Rubin*, Lorelei A. Mucci, Francesca Demichelis, Ove Andrèn, Sunita Setlur, Yujin Hoshida, Rameen Beroukhim, Yudi Pawitan, Robert Kim, Katja Fall, Hans-Olov Adami, Philip W. Kantoff, Swen-Olov Andersson, Todd Golub and Jan-Erik Johansson
US-Sweden Prostate Cancer Collaborative
The Dana Farber Harvard Prostate Cancer SPORE, USA, in collaboration with Örebro University Hospital, Örebro Karolinska Institutet, Stockholm, Sweden
**Brigham and Women's Hospital, Boston, MA, USA*

Prostate cancer causes considerable death and morbidity, yet many men harbor tumors that are indolent. Thus, some men receive unnecessary treatment, while others die of the disease despite aggressive therapy. In recent years, considerable effort has been devoted to identifying molecular markers to predict prognosis, without significant clinical impact. To address this question, we have assembled a multidisciplinary team of prostate cancer researchers from the US and Sweden. Our overarching goals are to identify and validate molecular signatures of indolent and aggressive prostate cancer that can be translated into clinical practice. To test and validate the molecular signature, we have assembled a large population-based natural history cohort of men with localized prostate cancer, consisting of 1,498 Swedish men with cancer [T1/2, N0, MX], diagnosed between 1977–1999 whose initial management strategy was watchful waiting. Formalin-fixed paraffin embedded (FFPE) archival tumor tissue at diagnosis is assembled for the entire cohort. Nationwide registers allows complete and long-term follow-up for prostate and all-cause mortality, and 241 of the men have died of prostate cancer through 2003. Moreover, a substantial proportion of men have long-term (> 10 years) disease-free survival, which affords considerable power to detect a signature of indolent disease. We will present our overall strategy of applying novel high throughput technologies to this unique clinical data set as well as data from one project, the validation in the Swedish watchful waiting cohort of a 12-gene model of aggressive prostate cancer evaluated by immunohistochemistry from an outcomes tissue microarray developed for this collaboration. The results suggest a molecular signature that can distinguish men with aggressive and indolent disease, over and beyond current clinical parameters.

Peptide-Linked Nanodevices for Biomarker Detection

Elizabeth Singer, Kristofer Munson, Jarrod Clark, Laura Crocitto, Timothy Wilson and Steven S. Smith
City of Hope National Medical Center, Duarte, CA, USA

We have used synthetic DNA Y-Junctions as fluorescent scaffolds for EcoRII methyltransferase-thioredoxin (M.EcoRII-Trx) fusion proteins. Unlike the 4-Way Holliday junction even though the Y-junction has symmetry, it is stable because it is not capable of branch migration via Watson-Crick base pairing. Covalent links between the DNA scaffold and the methyltransferase were formed at preselected sites on the scaffold containing 5FdC. The resulting self-assembling thioredoxin-targeted nanodevice was found to bind selectively to certain cell lines but not to others. Moreover, preliminary studies suggest that prostate tumor tissue gives stronger generalized fluorescence than normal tissue with the device.

The fusion protein was constructed so as to permit proteolytic cleavage of the thioredoxin peptide. Proteolysis with thrombin or enterokinase effectively removed the thioredoxin domain from the nanodevice and extinguished cell line specific binding as measured by fluorescence. The ability of the fused protein to selectively target the nanodevice to certain tumor cell lines suggests that this approach may serve as an adjunct to immunohistochemical methods in tumor classification.

Comprehensive DNA Methylation Mapping from Trace Human Specimens

Weiguo Han[a], James G. Herman[b] and Simon D. Spivack[a]
[a]*Wadsworth Center, New York State Department of Health, NY, USA*
[b]*Johns Hopkins Oncology Center, Baltimore, MD, USA*

A tag-modified bisulfite genomic sequencing (tBGS) method was developed for simplified evaluation of DNA methylation sites, employing direct cycle sequencing of PCR products at kilobase scale, in exfoliated cells and exhaled breath, as well as more conventional human specimens. The method avoids the need for conventional DNA fragment cloning; it entails subjecting bisulfite-modified genomic DNA to a second-round PCR amplification employing GC-tagged primers. Qualitative results from tBGS closely correlated those from conventional BGS ($R = 0.935$, $p = 0.002$). In application, the inter-tissue and inter-individual CpG methylation differences in promoter sequence for two genes, *CYP1B1* and *GSTP1*, were then explored across four human tissue types (peripheral blood cells, exfoliated buccal cells, paired nontumor-tumor lung tissues, exhaled breath condensate), and two lung cell types in culture (normal NHBE and malignant A549). Predominantly conserved methylation maps for the two gene promoters were apparent across donors and tissues. At any given CpG site, variation in the degree of methylation could be determined by the relative height of C and T peaks in the sequencing trace. Methylation maps for the *GSTP1* promoter diverged between NHBE (un-methylated) and A549 (completely methylated) cells in a previously unexplored upstream region, correlating with a 2.7-fold difference in GSTP1 mRNA expression ($p < 0.01$). Examples of its use in exhaled breath condensate samples from human subjects for lung *p16* promoter methylation are presented. The tBGS method simplifies detailed methylation scanning of kilobase-scale genomic DNA, facilitating more ambitious genomic methylation mapping studies, and trace DNA biomarker applications.

Development of Multiplexed Immunoassay Panels for Human Growth Factors and Growth Factor Receptors: bFGF, sFlt-1, PlGF, VEGF, KDR and c-Kit

Martin Stengelin, Anu Mathew, Selen A. Stromgren, Abrehet Abdu, Eli N. Glezer, Paul Grulich, John Joern, James L. Wilbur and Jacob N. Wohlstadter
Meso Scale Diagnostics, Gaithersburg, MD, USA

Growth factors and growth factor receptors are targets for cancer therapy and potential biomarkers to monitor disease progression. Electrochemiluminescence-based multiplexed immunoassay panels were developed for simultaneous measurement of multiple analytes per well in a 96-well format. Panel 1 detects the low-abundance analytes – *Basic Fibroblast Growth Factor* (bFGF), *Placental Growth Factor* (PlGF), *Vascular Endothelial Growth Factor* (VEGF), and *soluble VEGF Receptor 1* (sFlt-1 $\equiv$ VEGFR1), and was optimized for a 25 μL sample (serum or EDTA plasma). Panel 2 detects the more abundant analytes – *soluble VEGF Receptor 2* (KDR $\equiv$ VEGFR2) and *soluble Stem Cell Factor Receptor* (c-Kit), and was optimized for 50 μL of a 50-fold diluted sample.

The assay format is simple: diluent and sample are added to blocked and washed plates, and after a two-hour incubation with agitation, plates are washed, and detection antibody reagent is added. After a second two-hour incubation, plates are washed and read on a MSD SECTOR^{TM} Imager 6000 instrument (throughput of one plate per minute).

The lower and upper limits of the assay ranges in the following table represent the analytical sensitivity and the highest calibrator level, respectively. The linear range extends substantially beyond the highest calibrator level. Intra-plate CVs were approximately 4–8%. The assays are sensitive enough to measure these biomarkers in normal samples, and the dynamic range extends well beyond the elevated levels expected in disease states.

Analyte	Assay range	Analyte concentration in normal pooled serum and plasma samples (not paired)	
		Serum	EDTA Plasma
bFGF	1–9,000 pg/mL	< 1 pg/mL	7 pg/mL
sFlt-1	8–9,000 pg/mL	63 pg/mL	201 pg/mL
PlGF	1–9,000 pg/mL	13 pg/mL	16 pg/mL
VEGF	9–9,000 pg/mL	31 pg/mL	148 pg/mL
KDR	0.8–750 ng/mL	31 ng/mL	28 ng/mL
c-Kit	7–7,500 ng/mL	165 ng/mL	140 ng/mL

Each analyte in the multiplexed panels is measured accurately even in the presence of a high abundance of other analytes, as demonstrated in an experiment where an elevated concentration of one analyte at a time was spiked into a normal serum sample. Spike recovery and dilution linearity were in the range of 80% to 120%. In conclusion, multiplexed assays for simultaneous measurement of growth factors and growth factor receptors were successfully developed and validated.

Chromoendoscopic Colonoscopy Detects More Adenomas than Conventional Colonoscopy: A Randomized Trial of Back-to-Back Colonoscopies[1]

Elena M. Stoffel, David H. Stockwell, D. Kim Turgeon, Dan Normolle, Missy Tuck, Norman Marcon, John Baron, Robert Bresalier, Nadir Arber, Sapna Syngal and Dean Brenner
Brigham and Women's Hospital, Boston, MA, USA

Background: Conventional colonoscopy, currently the gold standard for the detection of colorectal neoplasia, misses some neoplastic lesions. Studies suggest that some flat adenomas may have high malignant potential. This EDRN-funded study was designed to 1) test whether application of contrast dye (chromoendoscopy) increases the sensitivity of colonoscopy for detecting adenomas 2) assess the prevalence of flat adenomas and collect tissue specimens for biomarker research. We present our findings from Aim 1.

Aim: To compare the efficacy of chromoendoscopy vs. standard colonoscopy for detecting adenomas, taking into account the prolonged inspection time of chromoendoscopy.

Methods: Fifty subjects with a personal history of sporadic colorectal cancer or adenomatous polyps underwent tandem colonoscopies at one of 5 study centers of the Great-Lakes New England Consortium of the Early Detection Research Network. The first exam for each subject was a "standard" colonoscopy with removal of all polyps found. The second exam was randomly allocated to be either pan-colonic indigo-carmine chromoendoscopy or conventional standard colonoscopy with intensive inspection lasting $\geqslant$ 20 minutes. Size, histology, and numbers of polyps detected on each exam were recorded.

Results: Seventeen of 50 (34%) subjects had a total of 40 adenomas detected on the initial conventional colonoscopy; 19 (48%) adenomas were found in subjects in the chromoendoscopy arm and 21 (52%) in jects in the chromoendoscopy arm and 21 (52%) in

those assigned to intensive inspection. Of the 27 subjects randomized to chromoendoscopy, 12 (44%) were found to have additional adenomas on second exam, 7 of these did not have adenomas on the initial exam. Among the 23 subjects randomized to intensive inspection, 4 (6%) had adenomas found on the second exam ($p = 0.07$), yielding a total of 5 additional adenomas. In the chromoendoscopy group 38 adenomas in total were detected; 19/38 (50%) adenomas were found on the second exam, as compared with 5/26 (19%) adenomas in the intensive inspection group ($p < 0.01$). Ten of the 24 adenomas missed on first colonoscopy were characterized as "flat" by predefined criteria. Of the 19 additional adenomas found during chromoendoscopy, 16 were located in the right colon versus two out of five for intensive colonoscopy. On average, polyps found on first colonoscopy were larger (3.74 $\pm$ 3.12 mm) than on second colonoscopy (2.39 $\pm$ 1.25 mm). Average inspection time was 29.7 minutes in the chromoendoscopy group, as compared with 20.4 minutes for the intensive inspection group. In multivariable analysis, the use of chromoendoscopy remained a significant predictor for detecting greater numbers of adenomas.

Conclusions: Chromoendoscopy detects more adenomas missed by standard colonoscopy than intensive inspection. Because as many as half of colonic adenomas may be missed by conventional colonoscopy, pan-colon chromoendoscopy may increase the yield for neoplastic lesions. Additional study of molecular characteristics of small and flat adenomas may help ascertain the clinical significance of these lesions.

[1]Supported by NCI grant CA 86400.

Incidence of Detecting Mutated K-ras DNA in Urine, Plasma and Serum from Patients with Carcinoma or Adenomatous Polyps

Ying-Hsiu Su[a,b], Mengjun Wang[b], Dean E. Brenner[c] and Timothy M. Block[b]
[a]Drexel University College of Medicine, Philadelphia, PA, USA
[b]*Department of Biochemistry and Molecular Pharmacology, Thomas Jefferson University, Doylestown, PA, USA*
[c]*Departments of Internal Medicine and Pharmacology, University of Michigan Medical Center, Ann Arbor, MI, USA*

Our previous studies demonstrated that urine contains DNA derived from tumor tissue from the circulation (Su et al., JMD 2004), suggesting that urine DNA has the potential for cancer detection. In this study, the incidence of detecting mutated K-ras DNA in body fluid (serum, plasma, and urine) from 20 patients with detectable codon 12 of the K-ras gene mutation in their colorectal disease tissue was compared. When DNA derived from 10 μl of body fluid was used in each mutation assay, the frequency to detect mutated K-ras DNA was comparable among serum, plasma, and urine. However, when DNA derived from 200 μl body fluid was used in the assay, the incidence of detecting mutated K-ras DNA in urine was significant higher (95%) than that of serum (35%) or plasma (40%) with $p < 0.0005$ as determined by the Fisher Exact 2-tailed test. The concentration of DNA in each body fluid was comparable between urine and serum, but the DNA concentration of plasma was significantly lower than that of urine and serum ($p < 0.05$). The size distribution of tumor derived DNA in the population of urine DNA was determined by agarose gel fractionation and was followed by the K-ras mutation assay, which found that mutated K-ras DNA was concentrated in the molecular weight fraction of less than 700 bp. The use of urine is advantageous because it is non-invasive and a larger volume is available for collection making it compelling to explore its application in clinical use.

Early Detection of Breast Cancer Using High-throughput Cloning of Tumor Antigens and Detection on Protein Microarrays

Jerzy Wojciechowski[a], Madhumita Chatterjee[a], Saroj Mohapatra[a], Bin Ye[a], Kathryn Carolin Amirika[a], Nancy Levin[a], Judith Abrams[a], Sorin Dragici[b] and Michael A. Tainsky[a]
[a]*Program in Molecular Biology and Human Genetics, Wayne State University School of Medicine/Barbara Ann Karmanos Cancer Institute, Detroit, MI, USA*
[b]*Department of Computer Science, Wayne State University, Detroit, MI, USA*

When cancer is identified at the earliest stages, the probability of cure is very high and therefore diagnostic screening tests that can detect these early stages are crucial. Efforts toward the development of early detection assays for cancers have traditionally depended on single biomarker molecules. Current technologies have been disappointing and have not resulted in screening tests suitable for clinical practice. The goal of this project is to detect antibodies that are produced by pa-

tients in reaction to proteins expressed in their breast tumors and use them as diagnostic biomarkers. The core technology of this project rests on research from the Tainsky lab in which he has developed a high throughput method to identify large numbers of epitopes that can be used to recognize the presence of cancer by detecting autoantibodies to tumor proteins in the serum of the test subjects. These biomarkers are cloned without a preconceived notion of their function. The essential features of the approach are acknowledging the heterogeneous nature of any specific kind of cancer, departing from the reliance on any single marker for disease detection, and using specialized bioinformatics techniques to interpret the results. The concept employs pattern recognition of multiple markers as a diagnostic rather than any single marker. In the discovery phase, the serum antibodies will be detected by screening large numbers of potential antigen targets on protein microarrays. The goal of this project is to detect antibodies that are produced by patients in reaction to proteins expressed in their breast cancers and use them as diagnostic and prognostic biomarkers. By a unique combination of techniques for cancer detection (microarray phage displayed auto-antigens), this study proposes to investigate a novel serum assay to detect and possibly predict outcomes of breast cancers. The serum reaction with large numbers of these antigens is to be detected in a highly parallel assay on protein microarrays. The principle is that we clone epitopes reacting with IgG in patients' sera and use them to detect antibodies in sera to discriminate between cancer and healthy subjects so as to detect disease prior to standard diagnosis. Our technology will provide an early detection test for breast cancer in asymptomatic women.

The dataset consisted of 98 serum samples including 48 stage I/II breast cancer patients and 50 healthy controls and 1737 antigens cloned by their binding to IgGs purified from two other breast cancer patients. A neural network was used for analysis of the data. The neural network used back-propagation to train and was part of WEKA machine learning software (Waikato Environment for Knowledge Analysis). The entire dataset was randomly divided into 2 groups. The larger group (66%) consisted of training examples for the neural net and the smaller group (34%) was used as an independent set of test cases for validation of training.

A t-test was performed three times, with progressively increasing the size of the clone set by lowering the p-value (0.01, 0.05, 0.10 respectively). The first test using a p-value $= 0.01$ selected 81 significant antigen clones and among 34 test cases there were only 6 misclassifications and an accuracy of 0.82. The second test using a p-value = 0.05 selected 254 antigen clones and among 34 test cases only 5 were misclassified. The accuracy improved to 0.85. In the third test using a p-value = 0.10 selected 368 antigen clones, and among 34 test cases only 2 were misclassified resulting in an overall accuracy of 0.94. Considering the heterogeneity of the disease and the small size of training data, the results seem very promising and justify further work on additional sera and markers.

Discovering Low Abundance Cancer Biomarkers: Balancing Depth of Coverage with Throughput and Confidence of Protein Assignment

Hsin-Yao Tang, Glenn Tan, Lynn Echan and David W. Speicher
The Wistar Institute, Philadelphia, PA, USA

Human serum and plasma are estimated to contain thousands of proteins, including proteins shed by all tissues and cell types in the body. The best candidate biomarkers capable of detecting early stage cancers are expected to be present at extremely low concentrations in blood; i.e., < 100 ng/ml. Even if higher abundance proteins are produced by tumors, their contributions are expected to be swamped by normal physiological fluctuations. We recently developed a 4-D plasma protein profiling strategy that detected far more proteins than alternative methods. Comparison of this dataset to plasma proteins with defined concentrations suggested that many of known proteins in the 1–100 ng/ml range were being detected. This strategy consists of major protein depletion, microscale solution IEF (MicroSol IEF) separation, 1-D SDS-PAGE, and nanocapillary reversed-phase HPLC separation of tryptic peptides with MS/MS analysis. Although this method could detect nearly 3,000 plasma proteins when HUPO criteria for high confidence peptide identification were used, throughput was extremely low and the false positive rate was unacceptably high. Therefore, we are pursuing two complementary approaches to further optimization of plasma proteome analysis.

First, we have developed data acquisition, database searching, and data interpretation strategies that yield individual peptide confidence assignments with false positive rates of < 2%, while retaining most of the true positive identifications of low abundance plasma proteins. One key factor is optimized data acquisition on a hybrid linear ion trap mass spectrometer to achieve sen-

sitive, rapid data acquisition with high mass accuracy capacity. Another key factor is use of partial tryptic constraints for database searches because many plasma protein false positives with full tryptic searches arise from large numbers of partial tryptic sequences caused by prior proteolysis in the initial sample. When full tryptic searches were performed, some of these spectra matched novel incorrect peptide sequences with good statistical scores, thereby greatly increasing the false positive rate. The effects of alternative data acquisition strategies on mass accuracy, number of proteins identified, and protein coverages were evaluated. False positive rates using different datasets and data filters were evaluated by searching combined forward and reverse databases.

Second, we are refining our basic multi-dimensional method to achieve high throughput, quantitative comparisons of patient samples, while retaining low ng/ml depth of protein coverage in human plasma. An automated method that requires less than 12 hours of instrument analysis time per proteome is being developed and tested. These improvements will significantly increase the confidence of our protein/peptide identifications, and allow us to increase the throughput of our analysis by at least 10-fold.

Pattern Detection and Cancer Diagnosis in Adult T-cell Leukemia Patients

Eugene Tracy[a], Haijian Chen[a], Dasha Malyarenko[a,b], Maureen Tracy[a,b], Liang Wei[a], Michael Trosset[a], Tina Bunai[a], Dennis Manos[a], Maciek Sasinowski[b], Richard Drake[c], Lisa Cazares[c], John Semmes[c] and William Cooke[a]
[a]*College of William and Mary, Williamsburg, VA, USA*
[b]*INCOGEN, Inc., Williamsburg, VA, USA*
[c]*Eastern Virginia Medical School, Norfolk, VA, USA*

We have applied our data processing techniques [1] to a major portion of the data from a 2004 SELDI-TOF protein expression profiling study of sera from Leukemia patients, conducted by EVMS [2]. After demonstrating that our signal analysis methods accurately reduce the spectral data to a small number of peak amplitude values, we have developed a number of visualization techniques to illustrate the patterns that can be used to classify many of the sample patients into one of the four patient groups: adult T-cell leukemia (ATL), HTLV carrier, HTLV-1 Associated Myelopathy/Tropical Spastic Paraparesis (HAM/TSP), and no disease. Our analysis verifies the earlier work showing the importance of the 11.7 kDa fragment of alpha trypsin inhibitor for diagnosing cancer [2], but also presents other marker candidates that are significant for distinguishing HTLV carriers and HAM/TSP from those with no disease. We demonstrate a variety of classifiers (trees, nearest neighbor classifiers, support vector machines, linear discriminant analysis, and neural networks) that use those visualization techniques for dimension reduction prior to classification, and we discuss the relative merits of each approach. We show that some of the marker candidates are also evident in the 2002 data set, after it has been aligned to the 2004 data set using our pre-processing techniques.

References

[1] Dariya I. Malyarenko et al., *Clinical Chemistry* **51**(1) (2005), 65–74.

[2] O. John Semmes et al., *Leukemia* **19**(7) (2005), 1229–1238.

Evaluation of Gene Expression Biomarkers for Cervical Intraepithelial Neoplasia[1]

M. Steinau[a], M.S. Rajeevan[a], D.R. Lee[a], M.T. Ruffin[b], I.R. Horowitz[c], L.C. Flowers[c], T. Tadros[c], G. Birdsong[c], M. Husain[d], S.D. Vernon[a] and E.R. Unger[a]
[a]*Centers for Disease Control and Prevention, Atlanta, GA, USA*
[b]*University of Michigan, Ann Arbor, MI, USA*
[c]*Emory University., Atlanta, GA, USA*
[d]*Wayne State University, Detroit, MI, USA*

Efforts to discover biomarkers for reliable early detection of cervical cancer have resulted in numerous candidate molecules that are dysregulated in neoplastic cells. However, their performance in clinical screening samples, such as routinely collected exfoliated cervical cell specimens remains to be demonstrated.

We used quantitative RT-PCR with a SYBR green assay to evaluate 40 candidate genes; 13 markers identified from our microarray data, 27 from current literature. Exfoliated cervical cell samples were collected from 93 women with CIN 3 or worse and 186 age, race and HPV matched (2:1) women without disease (CIN 0). Cervical disease status was based on the summary results of cytology, colposcopy and biopsy.

The samples were randomly divided into a training set (47 CIN 3+/94 CIN 0) and a test set (46 CIN 3+/92 CIN0). C_t values were normalized to an empirically established reference. The area under the curve (AUC) for each gene was calculated from C_t values for each sample set. We applied a low stringency cutoff [AUC > 0.6] to results from sample set 1 to identify genes with diagnostic potential to be evaluated in sample set 2 (test set).

Twelve genes had an AUC > 0.6 in the training set and were subsequently evaluated in the test set. Six genes, CLDN1 (Claudin1), MCM5 (mini-chromosome maintenance 5), MCM7, CDC6, MKI67 and SHCBP1 each gave an AUC > 0.6 in the second set as well. CLDN1 and MCM5 had the highest diagnostic value giving an AUC of 0.753 and 0.710 respectively for the combined sets.

As the markers were not highly correlated, we evaluated the possibility of a panel of five markers. The threshold for each marker was selected at the level of 90% specificity for CIN 3+. At this threshold for a positive test, 56 of 93 cases were positive for one or more of the five markers (60% sensitivity) as were 44 of the 186 controls (76% specificity).

These results indicate that gene expression in cervical cytology samples has potential to aid and improve routine screening, but additional markers and approaches to combining markers in panels is required.

[1]Supported by NCI's EDRN Interagency Agreement Y1-CN-0101-01.

Development of a Multiplexed DNA Methylation Assay for Prostate Cancer Detection

Shobha Varde, Joost Louwagie, Katja Bierau, Joseph Bigley, Jyoti Mehrotra, Tatiana Vener, Hsiling Chiu, Carlo Derecho and Abhijit Mazumder
OncoMethylome Sciences (OMS), Belgium and Durham, NC, USA
Veridex LLC, a Johnson and Johnson Company, Warren, NJ, USA

Introduction: Prostate cancer is the second leading cause of cancer-related deaths among men in the United States. The 25–30% false negative rate of initial biopsy screening calls into question which patients should undergo a follow up biopsy. Novel approaches for improved detection and prognosis in prostate cancer are needed. Evaluation of key cancer-related gene DNA hypermethylation using methylation-specific PCR (MSP) is one such approach. The use of a multiplexed, quantitative assay offers high evaluability of samples with limited DNA and is well suited for potential lab use.

Methods: OMS initially developed simplex assays run with the ABI 7900 as the readout platform for single gene determinations. More recently, Veridex constructed a homogeneous, multiplexed, Scorpion^{TM}-based assay for the quantification of promoter methylation levels for Glutathione-S-Transferase P1 (GSTP1), Adenomatous Polyposis Coli (APC), and Retinoic Acid Receptor $\beta2$ (RAR$\beta2$) on the Cepheid SmartCycler® II real-time instrument. A sample preparation protocol using the QiaAmp DNA Mini Kit^{TM} (Qiagen) was used to extract genomic DNA. Both simplex and multiplexed assays utilized ??-Actin as an indicator of DNA content.

Results: We present data from simplex assays performed on initial negative biopsy specimens from patients who underwent repeat biopsies which demonstrates the utility of methylation markers as a means to increase the Positive Predictive Value (PPV) of histopathology. A Scorpion based duplex assay measuring levels of GSTP1 and β-Actin demonstrated a sensitivity of 87% at a specificity of 100% using 142 formalin-fixed, paraffin-embedded prostatectomy and cancer-negative biopsy core samples, consistent with the published literature. Novel methods for multiplexed Scorpion analytical validation will be presented. Additionally, we present the design of an ongoing clinical study powered to detect an increase in the Negative Predictive Value (NPV) from an estimated 70% for histopathology alone to at least 85% in high-risk men with initial negative pathologic findings for prostate cancer.

Conclusions: A multiplexed, Q-MSP assay has been developed to measure critical gene hypermethylation levels for the detection of prostate cancer missed by standard histopathology. A potential application of such an assay in a prospective clinical study design is presented.

Chromosomal Aneusomy Detected by FISH in Sputum Predicts for Lung Cancer in Case-Control Study

Marileila Varella-Garcia, Aline P. Schulte, Chan Zeng, Holly J. Wolf, Fred R. Hirsch, Tim Byers, Tim Kennedy, York E. Miller, Robert L. Keith, Anna E. Barón and Wilbur A. Franklin
University of Colorado Health Science Center, Denver, CO, USA

Background: Survival rates for lung cancer are low mostly because patients have disseminated disease at diagnosis. Heavy cigarette smokers are known to be at high risk for lung cancer and constitute a target population for research in lung cancer prevention. There is an urgent need for development of non-invasive tests for monitoring and early detection of lung cancer in this population and sputum has long been considered a potential source of risk stratification among current and former smokers. We previously demonstrated that moderate or higher levels of cytologic atypia predict incident lung cancer in a cohort of heavy smokers with airflow obstruction and we now report the efficacy of the chromosomal aneusomy assay as a biomarker for cancer risk.

Methods: The study included 114 cases and 110 controls from the Colorado Sputum Screening Cohort Study who were matched on age, gender, and date of sample collection. Subject mean age was 67.4 ($\pm$ 8.1 years) and the female to male ratio was 1:3. All subjects had chronic obstructive pulmonary disease and $\geqslant$30 pack-years of tobacco use. Current smokers were 35% of the sample ratio and mean pack-years was 71.2 ($\pm$ 33.5). Chromosomal aneusomy was tested using the multi-target LAVysion probe (Abbott/Vysis).

Results: A total of 401 sputum specimens were assayed and the success rate was 83% in both case and control specimens. Slides were scanned for cytologic atypical epithelial cells characterized by large and irregularly shaped nuclei or patched chromatin staining by DAPI and the number of signals of each DNA target was determined in these atypical cells. An abnormal cell was defined as showing gain for $\geqslant$ 2 DNA targets or gain for $\geqslant$ 1 and loss for $\geqslant$ 2 DNA targets. Because tumor cells are expected to be rare in sputum, specimens were classified as abnormal when they showed $\geqslant$ 5% abnormal cells. The multi-target set showed the highest sensitivity (0.78) and specificity (0.95) rates in specimens collected within 12 months of lung cancer diagnosis. The individual probes EGFR, MYCC, 5p15 and CEP6 showed, respectively, decreasing sensitivity rates (0.78, 0.67, 0.62, and 0.29) and increasing specificity rates (0.84, 0.91. 0.86, and 0.95). Combinations of two specific probes (AND) or of any of two probes (OR) have not favorably impacted these coefficients. Proportion of abnormal sputum specimens was higher in squamous cell carcinoma than in adenocarcinoma or small cell carcinoma, both considering the set of specimens collected 12 months prior to disease diagnosis (92%, 75%, 60%) and all specimens (80%, 58%, 44%). Aneusomy had no significant association with cytologic atypia, which might indicate that molecular and morphological changes could be independent markers of tumorigenesis. Combining these tests improved sensitivity in specimens collected within 24 months of diagnosis (0.75% for only FISH to 0.80 for the combination) but decreased the specificity rates (from 0.92 to 0.77).

Conclusions: Chromosomal aneusomy in sputum was demonstrated in a nested case-control cohort to be a promising marker for prediction of lung cancer risk in heavy smokers with airflow obstruction. Evaluation of four DNA targets is more effective than any single marker or combination of markers, and the test has high sensitivity in patients with squamous cell carcinoma.

Structural and Numerical Chromosomal Abnormalities in Bronchial Cells from Heavy Smokers

Marileila Varella-Garcia, Lin Chen, Chan Zeng, Anna Baron, Fred Hirsch, Tim Kennedy, Robert Keith, York Miller and Wilbur A. Franklin
University of Colorado Health Science Center, Denver, CO, USA

Background: Cytogenetic alterations during lung carcinogenesis are incompletely understood. Aneuploidy is known to occur frequently in the airways of individuals at risk for lung cancer. However, numerical abnormalities alone may not accurately convey extent of chromosomal damage that may occur in the epithelium of smokers. Molecular karyotyping techniques permit complete chromosomal imaging of individual cells and facilitate the identification of masked and complex chromosomal abnormalities. To date, few studies have used these techniques to find critical abnormalities for initiation and progression of lung cancer.

Methods: Spectral karyotyping (SKY) was performed on non-malignant metaphase cells from bronchial cultures of 43 subjects from high-risk smokers without carcinoma, 14 patients with concurrent lung carcinoma and 16 never-smoker volunteers without lung carcinoma. High-risk smokers were selected on the basis of history of > 30 pack/year cigarette smoking, FEV1 > 70% of expected level and moderate dysplasia or worse on sputum cytology. Frequency and type of chromosomal abnormalities were compared in premalignant epithelium of high-risk smokers, cancer patients and never smokers.

Results: Seventeen (40%) of the high-risk smokers without carcinoma and 7 (50%) of the patients with carcinoma had clonal abnormalities while clonal abnormalities were not observed in never-smokers. Eight-two percent of the high-risk smokers and all of the carcinoma patients had at least one clonal or non-clonal abnormality while 75% of the never smokers had exclusively diploid cells (Chitest $p = 0.00002$). Clonal abnormalities observed in high-risk smokers and cancer patients included 20 chromosomal gains, 13 chromosomal losses, 8 partial losses, 3 balanced translocations and 3 unbalanced translocations. Clonal abnormalities occurring in more than a single individual included gains of chromosomes 5, 7, 8 and 18 and losses of chromosomes 10, 21 and 22. Non-recurring clonal and non-clonal partial losses and balanced and unbalanced translocations were frequent. To estimate the frequency of chromosomal abnormalities in individual specimens, we calculated the proportion of cells displaying numerical or structural anomalies/total number of cells evaluated which we refer to as the chromosomal abnormality index (CAI). Mean CAIs were 16%, 10% and 1% for cancer patients, high risk smokers and never smokers, respectively. The difference between high-risk smokers and never smokers was highly significant but the difference between cancer patients and high-risk smokers was not. Chromosomal gains observed by SKY were confirmed in interphase cultured cells or paraffin sections of biopsy specimens by FISH in 11 of 13 cases for which appropriate probes were available but chromosomal losses were not confirmed in any case.

Conclusions: Clonal and single cell abnormalities are frequent in bronchial epithelium of high risk smokers without carcinoma. Among these abnormalities were high frequency of chromosomal gains and an unexpected frequency of clonal balanced and unbalanced translocations. These results indicate a high frequency of chromosomal imbalance and damage in non-malignant bronchial epithelium before and in association with overt lung carcinoma and suggest that chromosomal missegregation and other chromosomal re-arrangements including translocations are common in during lung carcinogenesis before the development of malignancy.

Improved Prediction of PSA Biochemical Recurrence by Quantitative Nuclear Grade (QNG) Signature Compared to Pathology Findings Postprostatectomy[1]

Robert W. Veltri[a], Cameron Marlow[b], Danil A. Makarov[b], Michael C. Miller[c] and Alan W. Partin[b]
[a]Johns Hopkins University School of Medicine, Baltimore, MD, USA
[b]Baltimore, MD, USA
[c]Quakertown, PA, USA

Introduction: We calculated a nuclear morphometric signature, referred to as QNG, based upon variance of 40 nuclear morphometric descriptors (NMDs) that describe nuclear size, shape, DNA content, and chromatin texture in men with prostate cancer (PCa) that underwent radical prostatectomy (RP) and had long term follow-up. The objective was to evaluate the performance of QNG versus available routine pathological variables to predict PSA recurrence.

Methods: The NCI Cooperative Prostate Cancer Tissue Resource (CPCTR) tissue microarray (CPCTR-TMA) was prepared from RP cases treated in 1991–1992. A subset of the CPCTR-TMA cores were available from $n = 78$ cases ($n = 39$ non-recurrences and 39 PSA recurrences) with long term follow-up of about 12 years. Feulgen-stained nuclei were captured from two 0.20 mm spots for each case of the TMA using the AutoCyte[TM] Pathology Workstation. Multivariate logistic regression (MLR) was employed to calculate a QNG signature from 40 nuclear morphometric descriptors (NMDs) and Pathology variable statistical models. The MLR models to assess diagnostic performance, included a model constant, ß-coefficients, predictive indices from which predictive probabilities (PP) were derived for the two status groups. Kaplan-Meier plots were also performed for QNG and pathology variables.

Results: QNG was able to predict biochemical recurrence using eighteen (18) NMDs with a variable selection cutoff of $P_z = 0.15$ and the area of receiver operator characteristic curves (AUC-ROC) was **0.865** with a sensitivity of 92.3% and specificity of 59% and a accuracy of about 75.6% at a MRL cutoff of 0.30. Routine radical prostatectomy (RP) pathology yielded a AUC-ROC = **0.70** at a variable selection cutoff of $P_z = 0.15$ and the model retained only pathologic stage (p_Stage) and Gleason Sum Score yielded a sensitivity of 97% and specificity of 25.6% and a accuracy of 61.5%. When QNG and pathology were combined the MRL model had a sensitivity of 95% and a specificity of 61.5% and an accuracy of 78.2%, which was not statistically significantly that QNG.

Conclusions: In this NCI CPCTR-TMA ($n = 78$ PCa cases) we were able to predict of PSA biochemical recurrence using a nuclear morphometry signature (QNG), which was much improved compared to pathology information we had available. Next, we will need to apply add additional molecular biomarkers and also to obtain other PCa cases with similar follow-up to obtain validation of our QNG model.

[1]Funding Source: The Patana Research Fund and NCI-EDRN CA086323-06.

Quantitative Nuclear Morphometry Characterizes Differences in Feulgen Stained Nuclei Captured by Image Analysis from Primary Gleason Grading Patterns[1]

Robert W. Veltri[a], Cameron Marlow[b], M. Craig Miller[c], Masood A. Khan[d], Jonathan I. Epstein[b] and Alan W. Partin[b]
[a]*Johns Hopkins University School of Medicine, Baltimore, MD, USA*
[b] *Baltimore, MD, USA*
[c] *Quakertown, PA, USA*
[d] *UK*

Introduction: We assessed the alterations in structure of nuclei by Quantitative Nuclear Morphometry (QNM) based on nuclei captured from Gleason grading patterns 3, 4 and 5 of radical prostatectomy (RP) cases. The objective was to quantitatively compare normal prostate epithelia versus benign cancer-adjacent nuclei to prostate cancer of specific Gleason Grades (GG) from radical prostatectomy (RP) cases.

Methods: We used a tissue microarray (TMA) prepared from RP cases evaluated by a single pathologist (JIE). The prostate cancer (CaP) TMA cores were prepared from 20 GG-3, 9 GG-4, 10 GG-5 patterns, and 20 benign cancer-adjacent cases (All Gleason scores 3 + 3) selected from RP archival paraffin blocks. Feulgen-stained nuclei were captured from all four 0.2 mm spots for each case of the TMA (1100 objects each from GG-3; GG-4; GG-5; and benign, cancer adjacent nuclei) using the AutoCyte[TM] Pathology Workstation with QUIC DNA v1.10 software that includes morphometry and ploidy analysis. Next, we performed Multivariate logistic regression to calculate models that include a model constant, ß-coefficients, predictive indices and predictive probabilities (PP) for each pool of the three GG categories of nuclei compared to the benign cancer-adjacent nuclei. In addition, we plotted nuclei frequency distributions from GG 3, 4, and 5 patterns by using morphometric PPs solutions of all nuclei to illustrate shifts in trends of paired comparisons.

Results: QNM was able to objectively quantify, based on areas of receiver operator characteristic curves (ROC), differences between benign cancer-adjacent nuclei and GG-3 (ROC-AUC = 0.78) and an accuracy of 73%; GG-4 (ROC-AUC = 0.86) with an accuracy of 78% and GG-5 (ROC-AUC = 0.88) with an accuracy of 80%. Plots of the predictive probabilities (PP) of the three solutions compared to benign-cancer adjacent areas were all statistically significant ($p < 0.0001$). Frequency distributions of the individual cell nuclei PPs derived from primary Gleason grades 3, 4, and 5 demonstrated marked differences in PP patterns.

Conclusions: Utilizing benign cancer-adjacent prostate cell nuclei, we found significant differences in nuclear structure of Gleason grade 3, 4 and 5 patterns. Also, the nuclear morphometry PP distributions among these three GG may explain some of the biological and clinical variations seen in PCa. This is the first step in potentially objectively quantifying differences in Gleason grade nuclei that might used to eventually predict outcomes.

[1]Funding: The Patana Research Fund and NCI-EDRN CA086323-06.

Study Uptake in EDRN High Risk Registrants

Patrice Watson, Mary Benedetto and Henry T. Lynch
Creighton University School of Medicine, Omaha, NE, USA

Background: In 2001, The EDRN Clinical and Epidemiologic Center at Creighton University established the EDRN High Risk Registry (HRR). The Registry was founded to provide a pool of high risk individuals who could be recruited for EDRN studies. All persons recruited were judged to be at high risk for specific types of cancer because they were known carriers of cancer-associated mutation, most commonly in the BRCA1, BRCA2, MLH1, or MSH2 gene. Registrants complete a baseline questionnaire and yearly follow-up questionnaires. Here we report our first experience with recruitment from this pool, as we initiated the EDRN Longitudinal Serum Repository (LSB), a program of collection of annual serum and plasma specimens from persons at high risk for cancer. We also provide an update on the incidence of neoplasia among HRR members.

Methods: Members of the HRR were contacted my mail and invited to participate in the LSB. IRB-approved consent documents were included in the mailing.

Results: The HRR includes 375 persons. 268 (71%) are female. Most (46%) carry mutations in BRCA1. Other gene mutations represented, in order of frequency, are MLH1, BRCA2, MSH2, APC, CDKN2A, CDH1, and MYH. Seven weeks after the mailing of recruitment materials to 256 HRR members, 134 of them (52%) had returned signed LSB consent forms. 288 HRR members with follow-up information were evaluated for the occurrence of cancer (in-situ or invasive) and adenoma diagnoses, using Kaplan-Meier estimation of cumulative incidence. At 1, 2, and 3 years, the rates of cancer development were 4.5%, 7.6%, and 9.0%. The rates of developing either cancer or adenoma were 7.7%, 13.3%, and 18.1%.

Conclusions: EDRN investigators organizing prospective study of HRR members can expect recruitment rates of more than 50%, and high rates of cancer development among the recruited cohort.

Metrology for Cancer Biomarker: Affinity Analysis of Human HER2 with IgY

Yan Xiao[a], Gallya Gannot[b], Michael R. Emmert-Buck[b] and Peter E. Barker[a]
[a]*National Institute of Standards and Technology-NCI Cancer Biomarker Reference Laboratory, National Institute of Standards and Technology, Gaithersburg, MD, USA*
[b]*Advanced Technology Center Shady Grove, National Cancer Institute, Gaithersburg, MD, USA*

To improve quantitation of HER2 as cancer biomarker, we have generated novel avian IgY isotype antibody in cancer biomarker systems for comparisons with similar mammalian antibodies. IgY were generated against human HER2 synthetic polypeptide. IgY and IgG signals for HER2 were compared by immunohistochemistry (IHC), Western blotting and layered peptide arrays (LPAs). These studies suggest that although several mammalian antibodies for this target have been reported, metrology and quantitative comparisons of such affinity reagents in general are lacking. Here we demonstrate direct comparisons between mammalian and avian reagents with several methods. These results are directed at improved metrology necessary to validate both reagents, and subsequently the relationship between analyte concentration and patient outcomes in the clinic.

An Ultrasensitive FACTT Assay to Detect Melanoma Associated Biomarkers in Serum

X. Chen, H. Zhang, L. Schuchter, G. Acs, P. Van Belle, M.I. Greene and X. Xu
Departments of Pathology and Medicine, University of Pennsylvania, PA, USA

We have optimized a new antigen detection and quantification method that we term Fluorescent Amplification Catalyzed by T7 RNA polymerase Technology (FACTT). FACTT uses similar principles as the Enzyme-Linked Immunosorbent Assay (ELISA), however, in FACTT the detection antibody is directly coupled to a double-stranded DNA template that contains a T7 promoter to accommodate the attachment of the T7 RNA polymerase enzyme. The interaction of T7 leads to the production of RNA species that can be monitored by adding a fluorescent RNA intercalating dye. FACTT assay is developed in 96 or 384 well plates. It is an innovative isothermal quantitative high-throughput immunoassay platform. Our preliminary data demonstrated that FACTT assays consistently have at least a 1000-fold higher sensitivity than ELISA.

Malignant melanoma is a deadly disease. Melanoma cells express melanocyte lineage specific markers. Melanoma cells secrete soluble tumor markers, such as melanoma-inhibitory protein (MIA) and S-100beta. Tumor cell apoptosis and necrosis are common in malignant neoplasms even at an early stage. Our goals are to develop an ultrasensitive assay to detect early melanoma metastasis.

In this preliminary study, serum samples were collected from 4 patients with measurable metastatic melanomas and 4 healthy volunteers. We set up FACTT assays to detect tyrosinase and MIA. Pairs of antibodies were purchased from commercial sources. The capture antibody is coated in carbonate-bicarbonate buffer (pH 9.6) to 384-well plates at 5 μg/ml and at 20 μl/well overnight at 4°C. 1:100 dilution of serum in the amount of 20 μl per well, was added to the coated plate for a 1 hr incubation at room temperature. 20 μl of diluted biotinylated detection antibody (180 ng/ml, or an optimized concentration for each antibody) was used for each well and incubated at room temperature for 1 hr. Streptavidin and the biotin-DNA template (the amplification module, AM) were added sequentially at 5 μg/ml and 250 ng/ml, respectively, with a 1 hr room temperature incubation for each step. We washed the plate six times with PBST between each binding incubation. After excess AM and proteins were removed by washing, 20 μl of reaction mixture (containing 60 units of T7 RNA polymerase plus (Ambion), 1.25 mM NTP, 1x T7 buffer (Ambion)) was added to each well. RNA amplification is performed at 37°C for 3 hr. The RNA intercalating dye, RiboGreen, is added to the reaction mixture (20 μl, 1:200 diluted in the TE buffer supplied by the manufacturer) and the plates were read at Ex 485 nm/Em 535 nm in a TECAN SpectraFluor reader.

Our results showed that tyrosinase and MIA levels were significantly increased in patients with metastatic melanoma. Our data suggest that tyrosinase and MIA FACTT assays can be used to detect metastatic melanoma in serum. Additional studies are underway to confirm the findings.

ProMAT: A Bioinformatics Tool for Rapid Analysis of ELISA Microarray Data

Richard C. Zangar, Don S. Daly, Amanda M. White, Susan M. Varnum and Kevin K. Anderson
Pacific Northwest National Laboratory, Richland, WA, USA

Discovery technologies such as proteomics and DNA microarrays are identifying large numbers of proteins that have potential for detecting cancer. However, validating which sets of these proteins are clinically useful is a daunting task that requires the analysis of thousands of samples. Since current technologies have limited ability to quantify multiple proteins in large numbers of samples, we are developing a system for high-throughput protein analysis using enzyme-linked immunosorbent assay (ELISA) microarrays. As part of this process, we have developed a protein microarray analysis tool (ProMAT) specifically designed for generating standard curves and calculating protein concentrations for ELISA microarray experiments. ProMAT generates a tabular summarization of the data, a diagnostic image for each assay, and estimates the prediction errors for the sample data. This program is written in open-source code (R and JAVA) and is freely available at www.pnl.gov/statistics/ProMAT/.

Quantitative End-Point LATE-PCR Assays for Detection of LOH as a Biomarker

J. Aquiles Sanchez[a], Lawrence Wangh[a], Jesse Salk[b], Patricia Galipeau[b] and Brian J. Reid[b]
[a]*Department of Biology, Brandeis University, Waltham, MA, USA*
[b]*Divisions of Human Biology and Public Health Sciences, Fred Hutchinson Cancer Research Center, Seattle, WA, USA*

Our two laboratories are employing a new clinically compatible platform for the convenient and reproducible detection of LOH biomarkers in human cancers. Current methods for LOH detection are complex, expensive, and not sufficiently suited for routine clinical use. Our strategy, called Quantitative End-Point LATE-PCR (QE-LATE-PCR) permits robust and reliable LOH detection in small samples comprised of 1–100 premalignant cells. QE LATE-PCR assays are easy to perform in a single-tube format and are sensitive enough to detect chromosome loss in only a fraction of the genomes tested. We demonstrate the use of QE LATE-PCR for detection of LOH biomarkers in Barrett's Esophagus (BE), a precursor condition for esophageal adenocarcinoma (EA) and a model system for many cancers. A single center prospective (phase IV) study shows that a panel of three specific biomarkers (p16 LOH, p53 LOH, DNA content abnormalities – aneuploidy, tetraploidy) is highly predictive of EA risk in BE patients.

QE LATE-PCR identifies LOH by identifying SNP sites that are heterozygous in normal genomes but become hemizygous in genomes that have undergone LOH. Genotyping is based on the fraction of amplification products detected by a single hybridization probe at the end of the amplification reaction. The probe detects 50% amplification products in samples heterozygous for the probed allele, but either 100% or 0% of amplified products in hemizygous samples depending on whether the probed allele is retained following LOH or not.

Quantitative end-point genotyping is achieved through the combined use of LATE-PCR and mismatch tolerant probes. LATE PCR is a form of asymmetric PCR that generates single-stranded DNA products with high efficiency and specificity. The continued availability of single-stranded DNA products for hybridization at the end of LATE-PCR amplification permits product detection at multiple temperatures using mismatch tolerant linear probes. At a relatively high temperature, these probes preferentially hybridize to the fully complementary sequence of a particular SNP, but at a low enough temperature bind to all variants of that SNP. The ratio of fluorescence signals at the upper and lower temperature corrects for differences in product yield among replicates and reveals with 99.7% accuracy whether the sample in question possesses a normal diploid genome or an LOH genome due to loss of either chromosome.

LOH detection via QE LATE-PCR assays will greatly facilitate early identification of BE patients having the highest risk of developing EA. The same assays are available for rapid and reliable diagnostic of the many cancers and pre-malignant conditions in which LOH is a biomarker of neoplastic progression.

Kras^{G12D}, Cox-2 and Oxidative Stress

Gina DeNicola, Kenneth Yu, Ian Blair and David Tuveson
University of Pennsylvania, Philadelphia, PA, USA

Pancreatic ductal adenocarcinoma (PDA) is the most common pancreatic neoplasm and ranks fourth as a cause of death by cancer in the United States with a 5-year survival rate of only 3%. This is due to both the aggressive nature of the disease and the lack of specific symptoms and early detection tools. We have produced a mouse model of PDA by conditionally expressing a mutant endogenous *Kras*^{G12D} allele in the developing pancreas. Two-dimensional proteomic analysis was done to determine protein differences between primary mouse embryonic fibroblasts expressing *Kras*^{G12} and *Kras*^{G12D}, in an attempt to determine potential biomarkers of Kras activation. Despite the lack of measurable reactive oxygen species (ROS), proteomic analysis surprisingly revealed that fibroblasts display increased levels of multiple antioxidant response proteins following the expression of endogenous levels of KRas^{G12D}. Interestingly, the mRNA levels of many of these antioxidant response proteins were elevated, implicating a common process that coordinately regulates the transcription of this group of genes. Indeed,

Nrf2, a master regulator of antioxidant gene transcription, was elevated in whole cell lysates and nuclear extracts of cells expressing KRas^{G12D}. Nrf2 is known to be activated by many pathways including prostaglandin receptor signaling, and a chief enzyme responsible for prostaglandin synthesis, Cyclooxygenase type 2 (Cox-2), was present at higher levels in KRas^{G12D}-expressing cells and pancreatic tumors. Evidence for Cox-2 activation included increased levels of the lipid peroxidation byproduct thiadiazabicyclo-ONE-GSH-adduct (TOG) in KRas^{G12D}-expressing cells. TOG can arise from both non-enzymatic (ROS) and enzymatic (COX and LOX) lipid peroxidation, and the lack of measurable ROS in KRas^{G12D}-expressing cells supports the latter mechanism for TOG formation. Finally, ONE, which reacts with glutathione to produce TOG, is a reactive electrophile known to damage proteins, nucleic acids and other macromolecules. We propose that Cox-2 stimulates prostaglandin production in KRas^{G12D}-expressing cells and tissues that functions in an autocrine loop to promote proliferation and an anti-oxidant response to combat the presence of Cox-2 byproducts in cells. Cox-2 byproducts that are not detoxified, such as ONE, may further promote neoplasia by inducing genomic instability. Therefore, we plan to pursue the pharmacological and genetic inhibition of Cox-2 function in KRas^{G12D}-expressing cells to determine the importance of Cox-2 in the stimulation of proliferation and pancreatic cancer. In addition, we plan to examine these pathways in pancreatic cancer cells derived from PDA mice.

Application of Evidence Biochip Array Technology to Both Protein and DNA Analysis in Biological Samples

John Lamont
Randox Laboratories Limited, Antrim, Northern Ireland

Biochip array technology provides a platform that enable the simultaneous measurement of multiple markers in a clinical patient sample both in the fields of proteomics and genomics using miniaturized assay procedures with implications in the reduction of sample/reagent consumption and cost-effectiveness of the measurements. The core of the system is the biochip (9 mm^2) and represents not only the platform in which the capture molecules are immobilized and stabilised in pre-defined x, y coordinates defining microarrays of discrete test regions (DTRS) but is also the vessel were immunoreactions or hybridisation reactions are performed. Reactions are detected by chemiluminescence and the light emitted in each DTR on the biochip surface is simultaneously detected and quantified with a supercooled charged couple device (CCD) camera. The application of the dedicated analysers: the fully automated Evidence^R (FDA cleared) and the semiautomated Evidence Investigator^{TM} to this technology offers not only ease of use and higher sample throughput but as well superior control of the process and incorporation of system checks to assure results quality. The instruments incorporate dedicated software with capability to process, report and archive the multiple data generated for retrospective access.

Biochip array diagnostics is a valuable tool for research and clinical laboratories as is applicable to the detection of multiple analytes. This is illustrated here with excellent performance data for assays developed for the analysis of protein markers in human serum: tumour markers, adhesion molecules, cytokines and for DNA analysis in human stools: simultaneous detection of specific mutations within target genes in colorectal cancer (CRC).

Comparison of Prognostic Value of Molecular Markers of Colorectal Cancer Predicted by Proportional Hazards Regression and Linear Discriminant Analyses[1]

Sreelatha Meleth, William E. Grizzle and Upender Manne
Biomedical Statistics, Department of Medicine, and Department of Pathology, University of Alabama at Birmingham, AL, USA

Background: The majority of studies in cancer biomarker discovery use proportional hazards regression (PHREG) as a 'predictive' model but not as a 'classifier.' This study demonstrates the use of PHREG as a classifier. The quality of prediction of PHREG was compared to the prediction of a traditional classifier, linear discriminant analysis (LDA).

Methods: The PHREG and LDA models were built on a 491 CRC patient dataset comprised of demographic and clinicopathologic variables, including tumor TNM stage, and two molecular phenotypic markers (nuclear accumulation of p53 and Bcl-2 expression). The endpoint of prediction in these models was five-year post-surgery survival. The predictive ability of the models, with and without stages of the tumors as a variable, was compared using area under the *receiver operating characteristic* curves (AUC).

Results: The models were similar to each other in their predictive ability, with or without stage as a predictor variable (Table 1). The variables which emerged as significant in the model without the inclusion of tumor stage, were age with $p = 0.031$ [hazard ratio, HR $= 1.351$; 95% confidence internal (CI), 1.03–1.78], low Bcl-2 expression with $p = 0.02$ (HR $= 0.728$, 95% CI, 0.56–0.95), and tumor differentiation with $p < 0.0001$ (HR $= 1.947$; 95% CI, 1.40–2.70).

Table 1

Predicted probabilities (*test set*) at different cutoff values of probabilities obtained from PHREG and LDA

Values	Predicted outcomes of patients based on different predicted probability cutoff values					
	Cutoff = 0.5		Cutoff = 0.6		Cutoff = 0.7	
Models included TNM tumor stage together with other variables[a]						
True positives[b] (%)	83	65	46	74	46	74
True Negatives[c] (%)	27	52	54	49	54	49
AUC[d]	0.74	0.74	0.7	0.7	0.67	0.69
Models without including TNM tumor stage with other variables[a]						
True positives[b] (%)	69	71	59	73	35	73
True Negatives[c] (%)	68	63	70	54	82	54
AUC[d]	0.62	0.63	0.66	0.68	0.50	0.68

[a]Variables (age, tumor differentiation, Bcl-2 expression and p53[a,c]) were selected using iterative sampling (bootstrapping). Procedure repeated 1000 times. The variables that occurred in at least 500 of the 1000 lists were used in both models; [b]Proportion of individuals for whom the predicted outcome of death with in 5 years was right in the test set; [c]Proportion of individuals for whom the predicted outcome of survival beyond 5 years was right in the test set; [d]Proportion of individuals for whom the predicted outcome of death with in 5 years was right in the test set.

Conclusions: The findings of this study have demonstrated the usefulness of PHREG models in building classifier and the predictability of PHREG was comparable to LDA logistic regression. These findings also suggest that it might be possible to use Bcl-2 expression as a molecular marker to predict the patient prognosis when the information on tumor stage is not available.

[1]This work is supported in part by funds from the NIH/NCI (RO1-CA98932-01)[4] and the Early Detection Research Network (U24-CA086359).[3]

MALDI-TOF Analysis of Serum Peptides Associated with Hepatocellular Carcinoma

H.W. Ressom[a], S.A. Varghese[a], L. Goldman[a], A. Wang[a], F. Seillier-Moiseiwitsch[a], J. Liao[a], Y. An[a], E. Orvisky[a], S.K. Drake[b], G.L. Hortin[b], C.A. Loffredo[a], M. Abdel-Hamid[c], I. Gouda[d] and R. Goldman[a]

[a]*Department of Oncology, Lombardi Comprehensive Cancer Center, Georgetown University, Washington, DC, USA*

[b]*Department of Laboratory Medicine, Clinical Chemistry Service, NIH, Bethesda, MD, USA*

[c]*National Hepatology and Tropical Medicine Research Institute, Cairo, Egypt*

[d]*National Cancer Institute, Cairo, Egypt*

Introduction: Increasing incidence of hepatocellular carcinoma (HCC) in the US has been associated with hepatitis C (HCV) viral infections. We report a study of HCC in Egypt, a country with an epidemic of HCV and HCC. The goal of our study is to identify serum peptides associated with HCC for early detection and improved classification of the disease.

Methods: Serum samples were obtained in collaboration with NCI, Cairo, Egypt. Controls were recruited at the orthopedic fracture clinic and were matched to cases on gender, age, and residence (urban vs rural). We developed MALDI-TOF/TOF methods for analysis of serum peptides enriched by denaturing ultrafiltration and fractionation on magnetic beads. We compared 264 peptides by TOF-MS analysis of 78 HCC cases and 72 controls in the 0.8–5 kDa mass range identified, a subset of which was identified by TOF/TOF sequencing. Using newly developed computational methods, we selected 6 peptides that classify the disease with 100% sensitivity and 91% specificity in an independent set of 50 samples. Logistic regression analysis showed that each of the six peptides is significantly associated with HCC. Odds ratios for three peptides increased in HCC range from 1.4 to 2.8; odds ratios of three peptides decreased in HCC range from 0.4 to 0.7. Association of the biomarker-candidates with HCC is not substantially altered by age, gender, and viral infections. The peptides distinguish stage I and II tumors and distinguishing HCC patients from patients with cirrhosis in a pilot comparison ($n = 50$).

Conclusion: Using novel analytical methods, we identified six peptides that identify HCC with high prediction accuracy. A combination of six markers significantly improves the prediction accuracy of individual markers. These peptides should be useful in examining progression of chronic hepatitis C viral infection to malignancy. Development of a multiplex TOF-MS assay for quantification of the peptides is under way.

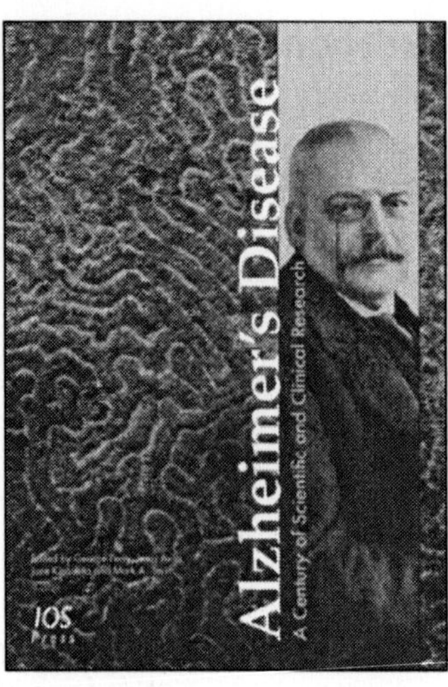

Alzheimer's Disease: A Century of Scientific and Clinical Research

Edited by: G. Perry, J. Avila, J. Kinoshita and M.A. Smith
July 2006, 468 pp., hardcover
ISBN: 1-58603-619-x
Price: US$150 / €120 / £82

This publication is a landmark work commemorating the centennial of Alois Alzheimer's discovery of what would be known as Alzheimer's disease (AD). The centennial of Alois Alzheimer's original description of the disease that would come to bear his name offers a vantage point from which to commemorate the seminal discoveries in the field. It traces how the true importance of AD as the major cause of late life dementia ultimately came to light and narrates the evolution of the concepts related to AD throughout the years and its recognition as a major public health problem, with an estimated 30-40 million people affected by AD today.

To identify the breakthroughs, the editors have used citation analysis, landmark papers identified by current researchers, and drew upon their own experience and insights. This process took into account the perspectives of individuals who recall the impact of findings at the time they were made, as well as of scientists today who have the advantage of hindsight in weighing the lasting influence of these findings. Because modern AD research was triggered by the seminal work of Tomlinson, Blessed, and Roth some four decades ago, it is particularly fortunate that the vast majority of these milestone authors are still with us.

-ORDER ONLINE AT WWW.IOSPRESS.NL-
Select the title of your choice and click on *order online*

IOS Press is a rapidly expanding Scientific, Technical, Medical and Professional publishing house focusing on a broad range of subject areas, such as; medical science, healthcare, telecommunication, artificial intelligence, information and computer science, parallel computing, physics and chemistry, environmental science, and other subjects.

IOS Press

IOS Press	**IOS Press, Inc.**	**Gazelle Book Services Ltd**
Nieuwe Hemweg 6B	4502 Rachael Manor Drive	White Cross Mills
1013 BG Amsterdam	Fairfax, VA 22032, USA	Hightown
The Netherlands	Tel. +1 7003 323 5600	Lancaster LA1 4XS
Tel.: + 31 20 688 3355	Fax: +1 703 323 3668	United Kingdom
Fax.: + 31 20 687 0039	E-mail: iosbooks@iospress.com	Tel.: +44 1524 68765
E-mail: market@iospress.nl		Fax: +44 1524 63232
URL: www.iospress.nl		E-mail: sales@gazellebooks.co.uk
		URL: www.gazellebooks.co.uk

Visit our website for more information or online ordering:
www.iospress.nl